D1503655

PSYCHIATRIC DISORDERS IN ADOLESCENTS

PSYCHIATRIC DISORDERS IN ADOLESCENTS

Richard W. Hudgens, M.D.

Professor of Clinical Psychiatry
Washington University School of Medicine
Saint Louis, Missouri

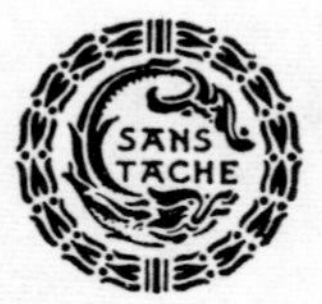

THE WILLIAMS
& WILKINS COMPANY / BALTIMORE

The Williams & Wilkins Company
428 E. Preston Street
Baltimore, Md. 21202, U.S.A.

Made in the United States of America

Library of Congress Cataloging in Publication Data

Hudgens, Richard W
Psychiatric disorders in adolescents.

1. Adolescent psychiatry. I. Title.
[DNLM: 1. Mental disorders—In adolescence. WS462
H884p 1974]
RJ503.H8 616.8'9 74-3431
ISBN 0-683-04217-3

Composed and printed at the
WAVERLY PRESS, INC.
Mt. Royal and Guilford Aves.
Baltimore, Md. 21202, U.S.A.

TO THE MEMORY OF
ROBERT WATTS HUDGENS

ACKNOWLEDGMENTS

The study of adolescents reported in this book was carried out in the Department of Psychiatry of the Washington University School of Medicine. Earlier clinical investigations by members of the department, as well as their advice during this project, provided encouragement and excellent examples to follow. In this regard, I am especially grateful to Dr. Eli Robins, Professor and Head of the Department of Psychiatry, whose leadership has been chiefly responsible for the spirit of free inquiry which prevails among faculty and trainees in the department; Dr. Samuel B. Guze, Professor of Psychiatry; Dr. George Winokur, now Chairman of the Department of Psychiatry at the University of Iowa School of Medicine; and to Dr. Lee Robins, Professor of Sociology in Psychiatry at Washington University.

Five psychiatric residents, in training at the time of the study, participated with me in interviewing the adolescent subjects and their relatives: Drs. E. Kent Stevenson, Carl P. Held, Charles H. Meredith, Ramnik G. Barchha, and James R. Morrison. Dr. Stevenson also took part in the early stages of data analysis. The laborious tasks of interview coding and data analysis were carried out by Mrs. Miriam E. Hendrix and Miss Dianne L. Carr. And Mrs. Sue Lavin typed the rough and final manuscripts, deciphering my handwriting in the process.

I am most appreciative of the intelligence and help of all these people whose hard work made the book possible. And I especially thank the teenagers and their families, who were the subjects of this work and who cooperated in the research project at a time of great difficulty in their lives.

This work was supported in part by the following U.S.P.H.S. Grants: MH-14634, MH-05804, MH-13002 and MH-10356.

TABLE OF CONTENTS

TABLE OF CONTENTS

INTRODUCTION

This book is about psychiatric illness in a group of young people who were sick enough to be hospitalized at least once before they were 20 years old. It deals with psychopathology in the broad sense of the word: not only with the clinical manifestations of psychiatric illnesses, but also with their courses over time, with associated interpersonal, sociologic, and scholastic factors, and with psychiatric and social disturbances in the families of patients. A final chapter is concerned with the principles of therapy for various psychiatric illnessess in adolescents.

One main purpose of the book is to provide a more complete and systematic classification and description of psychiatric disorders among teenagers, to the end that such patients may be better understood and more effectively treated. Another purpose of this work is to provide the basis for a comprehensive follow-up study, from adolescence well into adulthood, of persons with the early onset of psychiatric illness. Such a longitudinal investigation should yield information about the early and perhaps atypical manifestations of common syndromes, for example, alcoholism and depression, as well as a clearer definition of the nature and development of those "personality disorders" which have not yet been well described or classified. Furthermore, a prospective study with systematic attention to the chronology of positive and negative psychiatric, sociologic, and medical features will identify factors which are important predictors of various outcomes. This is a subject about which there are many theoretical assertions but too few reliable data in psychiatry.

In preparation for this book, 220 adolescents were studied: 110 psychiatric inpatients and 110 controls who were inpatients on pediatric, medical, or surgical services and who had never been hospitalized for psychiatric disorders. The syndromes and special problems which this work considers in detail were those found in the subject population. These young people were admitted to a large university medical center where the primary emphasis was on diagnosis and treatment of acute disorders or acute exacerbations of chronic disorders requiring relatively brief periods of hospitalization. Accordingly, among the psychiatric patients there was a predominance of affective syndromes, acute psychoses, and behavior disorders for which psychiatric hospitalization (rather than placement in a correctional institution) was deemed justifiable. A substantial proportion (41%) of the psychiatric inpatients in this investigation had made suicide attempts at some time in their lives.

Because of those characteristics of the patients studied, the book does not deal at length with some of the disorders commonly found among psychiatrically ill adolescents, such as chronic brain syndromes, mental deficiency, or severe and repetitive criminal behavior. And because this is a study of inpatients, this work does not discuss in depth those disorders for which teenagers are seldom admitted to a psychiatric hospital, for example, hysteria, anxiety neurosis, obsessive compulsive neurosis, phobias, sexual deviation, and relatively uncomplicated learning disorders.

Finally, this is not a book about adolescence as a time of life. One thesis of this work, based upon this and other systematic studies, is that in the majority of teenagers who are psychiatrically disturbed their "illnesses" are more important than their "adolescence." Nevertheless, the processes of physical, emotional, and social change of the teenage years may exert considerable influence on the form and course of the disorders, and the people treating adolescents must be familiar with these processes.

1

Methods of study

INTRODUCTION

The subjects of this study were adolescent inpatients on the psychiatric and non-psychiatric services of the Washington University Medical Center in St. Louis. The several hospitals comprising the Medical Center contain 1307 beds, including 104 in Renard, the psychiatric hospital. As the major site of treatment, research, and training for the Washington University School of Medicine, the Center is staffed by a large full-time and part-time faculty and by resident physicians in all specialties. Less than 5% of the patients are cared for on a charity or part-pay basis. Costs of the great majority are covered by patients and insurance companies. Emphasis is on the short and intermediate term treatment of people with acute disorders, or exacerbations of those chronic disorders which require relatively brief periods of hospitalization.

There are between 1500 and 1600 annual admissions to the psychiatric inpatient service of Renard Hospital and a 90 to 95% occupancy rate for the 104 beds. The average inpatient stays between three and four weeks. Patients are actively treated for their disorders and return to their families, schools, jobs, and outpatient treatment as rapidly as possible.

SELECTION OF PSYCHIATRIC INPATIENTS FOR STUDY

Before the start of our investigation, we decided to study 110 adolescent psychiatric inpatients, ages 12 through 19, so that at least 100 might be located at follow-up 10 to 12 years later. During the period of this study, from September 1, 1965 to February 27, 1968, there were 3814 admissions to the psychiatric service. Of these, 351 (9.7%) were admissions of patients who were from 12 to 19 years old. These 351 admissions were of 302 different adolescents, 265 of whom were admitted once and 37 twice or more during the study period.

The 110 adolescent psychiatric patients were selected in the following way: each day during the study period the author received a list of the names and ages of patients admitted to Renard Hospital on the previous day. Each patient from 12 through 19 years old was selected for investiga-

TABLE 1

Comparison of Adolescent Psychiatric Patients Selected for Study with Those Not Selected

	Patients Studied N = 110	Patients Not Studied N = 192
	%	%
Boy	40	46
Girl	60	54
White	87	86
Black	12	14
American Indian	1	0
Mean Age	16.50 years (S.D. 2.04)	16.98 years* (S.D. 1.92)

* Age distribution: $t = 2.11, p < .05$ (more younger patients in studied group).

tion if one of the physicians* involved in the study had time available for the long research interviews of the adolescent and a relative within two days of admission, before active treatment had altered the clinical picture. None of the psychiatric patients or their parents refused to cooperate.

Table 1 compares the 110 adolescents in the study with the 192 adolescents who were admitted to the psychiatric service during the period of investigation but not studied. There was an unintended bias in favor of selection of younger patients: a larger proportion of study patients (35%) than non-study patients (21%) were from 12 to 15 years of age. With regard to sex and race the psychiatric patients selected for study did not differ significantly from those not selected.

SELECTION OF CONTROLS

Control subjects for the psychiatric inpatients were selected during three study periods: February 1 to 27, 1968; May 1 to June 19, 1968; and July 1 to September 14, 1969. The following method was used: daily lists were obtained containing the name, age, sex, and race of each person admitted to a nonpsychiatric service of the Washington University Medical Center. From the information on these lists we identified prospective controls, each of whom matched a specific psychiatric patient for age, sex, and race. We then sought permission from each prospective control, his parents, and his physician for inclusion in a "study of teenagers in hospitals," if the patient had never been admitted to any hospital for psychiatric treatment (our only criterion for exclusion). As more and more controls were interviewed, the number of potential controls identified from each day's list diminished.

There were 730 patients ages 12 through 19 admitted to the non-psy-

* The author and five psychiatric residents, Drs. E. Kent Stevenson, Carl P. Held, Charles H. Merideth, Ramnik G. Barchha, and James R. Morrison.

chiatric services during the three study periods. Of these, 156 were identified as prospective controls. Fortuitously, none of them had ever been hospitalized for psychiatric symptoms. Of the 156, 46 were not interviewed: four because they were unconscious, three because their physicians refused permission, and 39 because they were discharged before the interviewer could reach them (usually within 48 hours of admission).

The remaining 110 were the control subjects in our study.* They differed from the 620 other teenagers hospitalized on non-psychiatric services during the study periods in that their mean age was six months greater, and a significantly larger proportion of the studied sample was white (84% *vs.* 74%). Since non-psychiatric patients who were discharged within two days of admission were more likely to be missed, even if selected as potential controls, such short-stay patients were under-represented in the final control sample.

It was felt to be more important that the controls resemble the psychiatric inpatients as closely as possible than that they be representative of teenagers in a general hospital sample. Thus, insofar as possible, the psychiatric patients and controls were selected to be alike, with the only intended difference to be that the latter group have no history of hospitalization for psychiatric disorder.

INTERVIEWS AND DATA COLLECTION

Each psychiatric patient and control received a research interview which required from one and a half to five hours, usually administered within 48 hours of admission. An interview requiring more than two hours was customarily divided between two appointments on consecutive days. The same research interview was separately administered to at least one relative, usually one or both parents, except in the cases of nine psychiatric inpatients. However, information from the families of those nine adolescents was gathered by the psychiatric residents and attending staff responsible for care of the patients, recorded in their hospital records, and used in this study. Thus there were 101 informant interviews in the cases of the 110 psychiatric inpatients. Both parents were interviewed in 17 cases, the mother in 65, the father in 12, spouse in four, another relative in one case, and a non-relative in two cases. Relatives were systematically

* Because of clerical errors in the admission lists from which the controls' age-sex-race categories were compiled, the psychiatric patient sample contained two more boys than the control sample, one more black patient, one more 15-year-old, two less 18-year-olds, and one more 19-year-old. An American Indian girl in the psychiatric sample could not be matched for race and was matched with a white girl of the same age in the control sample. These small differences between psychiatric patients and controls did not significantly affect the similarity between the two groups with respect to age, sex, and race.

interviewed for all 110 controls: the mother in 91 cases, father in seven, a sibling in two cases, spouse in seven, other relatives in two, and a non-relative in one case. Thus of the 211 informant interviews for psychiatric inpatients and controls, 201 were with a parent or spouse. The spouses of 11 of the 13 married subjects were interviewed.

The research interview contained both structured and unstructured parts and is detailed in Appendix I. Customarily, the interviewer began by requesting a spontaneous account of the events leading to admission, a history of past and present psychiatric and medical disorders, and a review of important circumstances in the patient's life, including his functioning in his family, school, and relevant interpersonal relationships. The history of past and present disorders and treatment or counseling was then explored systematically, with both positive and negative information recorded. Inquiry was then made about gestation and birth; growth and developmental histories; school and job histories in terms of performance and attendance, with specific inquiries about all lapses and impairments; legal and military history; parents' occupational and financial status; dynamics of family, school, and peer relationships; sexual development and activity; dates of birth and death (and cause of death) of all first degree relatives; history of psychiatric illness and suicide in near and remote relatives; the occurrence or absence of specified stressful, or otherwise important, life events; suicide thoughts, communication and attempts; and the use of alcohol and drugs. Each subject and informant was then questioned regarding the presence or absence of 110 psychiatric and medical symptoms. A symptom was scored as positive if it met the following criteria: (a) the symptom led the patient to go to a physician, or (b) the symptom was disabling, causing some degree of change in his life, or (c) the symptom led the patient on more than one occasion to take medication, or (d) the investigator believed the symptom should be scored as positive because of its unusual nature, persistence, or frequency. Every negative response was recorded as such. Every putatively positive response was investigated by further questions to see if it fulfilled one of the criteria listed above for positive scoring. If it did, the response was elaborated with regard to its quality, frequency, and chronology.

It should be emphasized that care was taken to record negative information—the absence of a symptom or of behavioral, scholastic, and interpersonal disruption. To understand the current clinical picture and provide the basis for a systematic follow-up study, it was as important to know which things did *not* occur as to know which things did occur.

To make it easier to locate the subjects at follow-up, the interviewer obtained the names and addresses of parents, spouse (if any), and at least two other adult relatives, perferably a man or married woman (whose name would not likely be changed during the follow-up interval).

After the subjects were discharged from the hospital their charts were examined and information recorded. At that time also the records of all previous admissions to hospitals in the Washington University Medical Center were examined and data recorded. Records were then requested from all schools and colleges ever attended by the subjects, from all physicians whom they had consulted, and from all hospitals where they had been treated at any time in their lives. Follow-up letters were sent to persons and institutions who did not respond to the first request. In all, school records were collected concerning 105 of the 110 psychiatric patients and 101 of the 110 controls. Medical records from physicians and hospitals outside the Medical Center were obtained for 68 patients and 72 controls.

Information from all sources was coded, punched on IBM cards, and analyzed. Three methods were used to test the statistical significance of differences between comparison groups: the chi-square method (using the Yates correction for small numbers when appropriate), the standard error of the difference between proportions, and the *t*-test.[1] A difference between samples were considered significant if the probability of its occurrence by chance was less than 5%.

REFERENCE

1. Hill, A. B. *Principles of Medical Statistics.* London, Oxford University Press, 1961.

2

Diagnosis

GENERAL CONSIDERATIONS

Diagnostic classification presents a greater problem in psychiatry than in other fields of medicine. One reason for this is that no biologic correlates have been discovered for most of the illnesses psychiatrists treat—disorders of thinking, mood, and behavior. Some chronic organic brain syndromes, such as general paresis, senile psychosis, and arteriosclerotic psychosis, are exceptions in this respect. But in most forms of delirium and in the psychiatric disorders commonly called "functional," physicians depend upon the history and observations of the patients' behavior and speech to make their diagnoses. No one knows, for example, the "essential" nature of schizophrenia, although the body's fluids and the brain have been examined extensively for clues since early in this century. There is, moreover, considerable disagreement among psychiatrists as to whether schizophrenia is only one disorder or several, and disagreement as to how it should be subdivided.

So the lack of biologic correlates or pathognomonic features in most psychiatric disorders has been partly responsible for the development of a plethora of diagnostic systems and non-systems. Disturbances of thought, mood, and behavior have been variously classified according to clinical picture, supposed etiology, or degree of social dysfunction. Some writers have even denied the scientific validity of classifying psychiatric syndromes at all, viewing diagnostic terms merely as society's epithets for deviant behavior.[1] The general state of uncertainty has led some psychiatrists to question the value of diagnosis, and to pay only lip-service to it, as when they are filling out insurance forms or completing hospital records.

In the United States, another reason for the under-valuation of the diagnostic process has been the widespread practice of studying individual patients intensively to the exclusion of studying the syndromes from which they suffer. In many American psychiatric institutions, it is the tradition that every case is formulated principally along psychodynamic lines, with emphasis on features of psychopathology, life history, and interpersonal relationships which are unique to that particular person. Paying attention to individual features in this way is necessary for psychotherapy and the general management of patients, but an *exclusive* emphasis on individual characteristics can be misleading, and harmful to patients.

On the other hand, there is considerable evidence, through clinical descriptions, follow-ups, and family studies, that psychiatric syndromes exist, although their causes are largely unknown, and that for certain syndromes (for example, manic-depressive illness, schizophrenia, hysteria) the diagnosis has more predictive value than the individual's psychodynamics. Not all patients can be confidently classified, but in studies done at the Washington University Medical Center we have found that at least three-quarters can be.[2, 3] At any rate, classification of a patient according to a well established syndrome, whenever it is possible, does not prevent a psychiatrist from giving proper attention to the case's uniquely individual aspects.

DIAGNOSTIC PROBLEMS IN ADOLESCENTS

Where adolescents are concerned, diagnostic classification presents even more problems, and is a more controversial subject than among adult patients. In studies done at Washington University and elsewhere, fewer teenagers than adults can be fitted with certainty into established diagnostic categories.[2, 4] One explanation for this may be that many of the adolescent psychiatric patients have not been sick long enough or often enough to have developed the longitudinal clinical features of established syndromes. For example, a diagnosis of "process" schizophrenia (chronic schizophrenia, as contrasted with a remitting "schizophreniform" disorder[5]) should not be made until the illness has persisted for more than just a few months. And an adolescent who is going to become an alcoholic might in his early teens manifest primarily impulsiveness, poor tolerance for stress, and difficulty getting along with people. He may not begin drinking heavily until later. It has also been suggested that some psychiatric disorders, for example depression, might show atypical clinical pictures when they appear in younger people.[6]

Another reason for the uncertain status of diagnostic classification among teenagers is a traditional view that the process of adolescence itself is psychopathologic. Support for this theory has been largely anecdotal, related to individual case reports and extrapolations from them. Recent systematic longitudinal studies of normal adolescents by Offer,[7] and of psychiatric patients and controls by Masterson,[8] help to refute such notions. Psychiatric impairment occurs only in a minority of teenagers, and this minority can be differentiated from the rest by the presence of emotional and behavioral symptoms which tend to persist over time or recur.

It is true that certain things occur only in the teenage years or occur much more frequently then than at other times of life: pubescence, maturing sexual responses, accelerated body growth, increased capacity for abstract reasoning, reorientation of peer-group associations including sexual relationships, increasing independence from parental authority, career decisions, and so forth. These processes and events are accompanied by emotional and behavioral changes, as are processes and events in childhood, young adulthood, middle life, and old age. But such changes are usually not psychopathologic, and when they are, the pathology cannot with certainty be attributed to the life events. In any case, adolescence itself is not psychopathologic, and psychiatric disability, if defined as the presence of social, emotional, cognitive, or behavioral impairment requiring treatment, does not occur more frequently in adolescence than in later life. It occurs *less* frequently, as has been demonstrated in epidemiologic surveys and in studies of psychiatric patients.

DIAGNOSTIC CLASSIFICATION IN THE CURRENT STUDY

Granted the difficulties involved in making psychiatric diagnoses and the impossibility of choosing a diagnostic system which will meet with the approval of all psychiatrists, systematic classification of psychiatric patients should always be attempted. In the present early stage of scientific clinical investigations in psychiatry, such classification may be as important as anything else. The definition of syndromes has been the foundation of the longitudinal clinical investigations and the pathologic, biologic, social, and family studies which comprise psychiatry's real body of knowledge and which can lead to more complete understanding of the nature, causes, treatment, and prevention of psychiatric disorders. Classification and subsequent studies in the above areas are as important for understanding psychiatric syndromes that may turn out to have predominantly experiential causes as for understanding those that have biologic origins, caused, for example, by genetic factors or by toxic substances entering the body. Thus it would seem desirable, both for purposes of research and for treating individual patients, that the psychiatrist use specific criteria for the diagnosis of each psychiatric syndrome. These criteria should not only describe the disorder in question, but also distinguish it from other disorders.

During the past three decades at the Washington University School of Medicine criteria for diagnosing the various psychiatric syndromes have been developed and validated through longitudinal clinical and family studies done in this Department of Psychiatry and elsewhere. Recently, Feighner et al.[9] published a paper setting forth these criteria. For our current study of psychiatric illness in adolescents, we used diagnostic criteria which were identical or very similar to those later appearing in the

Feighner paper. The specific criteria used in our study are listed in Appendix II.

An adolescent subject in our investigation was classified diagnostically only when his clinical picture and course conformed to the predetermined criteria for inclusion in a specific diagnostic category *and no other.* Diagnosis was restricted to those syndromes which had been shown to have characteristic and generally predictable courses over time on the basis of systematic longitudinal clinical and family studies. If a psychiatrically ill patient did not fit into such an established diagnostic group, or if, in spite of resembling other patients with a given diagnosis, he did not fulfill the criteria for that syndrome, he was called "psychiatric illness, undiagnosed." Diagnostic terms which have not acquired respectability through systematic studies were avoided: for example, adjectival labels, like "inadequate personality," or mere symptom descriptions masquerading as diagnostic terms, like "hypochrondriacal neurosis."

In this study, if a patient had more than one psychiatric disorder, the illness coming first in time was designated "primary," regardless of its relative importance, and the illness(es) of later onset was termed "secondary" ("tertiary," etc.). In cases with more than one diagnosis the disorder which was more disabling in the opinion of the investigator was designated the "principal disorder," regardless of whether or not it was "primary."

As mentioned above, subjects whose illnesses did not fit established diagnostic criteria were termed "undiagnosed." Among the undiagnosed group those whose disorders resembled (but did not quite fit) the clinical picture of established diagnostic groups, were subclassified: for example, "undiagnosed, most like depression," ". . . most like hysteria," etc. In the special case of patients who were undiagnosed because the investigators could not decide whether they had schizophrenia or a severe affective disorder, the term "schizoaffective" was used. The remaining patients, who could neither be classified as definitely or possibly belonging to an established diagnostic group, were called "undiagnosed, unclassified."

DIAGNOSES AMONG ADOLESCENTS IN THIS STUDY

Table 2 shows the distribution of psychiatric patients and controls among the various diagnostic groups. All but one of the psychiatric inpatients were psychiatrically ill, that is, socially impaired by disorders of thought, mood, or behavior. The exception was a 13-year-old girl who was admitted after a fainting spell. By contrast the controls had a lower incidence of psychiatric disorders, and such illnesses, when present, were milder than those of the psychiatric inpatients. Thirty-nine controls had psychiatric syndromes. Seven of these had *only* epilepsy (four) or mental deficiency (three) as psychiatric diagnoses. The other two of the six epileptic controls had functional psychiatric disorders in addition to

TABLE 2

Principal Research Diagnoses among Adolescent Psychiatric Inpatients and Controls

	Psychiatric Inpatients N = 110	Controls (Non-psychiatric Inpatients) N = 110
Depression	19	8
Mania	11	0
Schizophrenia	6	0
Antisocial Personality	7	2*
Epilepsy	0	6*
Mental Deficiency	1	3†
Organic Brain Syndrome	1	0
Alcoholism	1	0
Anxiety Neurosis	0	1
Anorexia Nervosa	1	0
Undiagnosed Psychiatric Illness:		
most like depression	14	13*
most like antisocial personality	7	3
most like hysteria	2	1
most like schizophrenia	1	0
between depression and other diagnosis	2‡	0
schizoaffective	7	0
unclassified	29	2
No psychiatric illness ever	1	71‖

* Two of the six controls with the principal diagnosis epilepsy had functional psychiatric disorder: one had an antisocial personality, making a total of three controls with that diagnosis; the other was "undiagnosed, most like depression," making 14 controls with that diagnosis. The remaining four epileptics had no psychiatric complications and are classified with the psychiatrically "well controls" in Chapter 3.

† None of the controls with mental deficiency had other psychiatric disability. They are classified in Chapter 3 with the psychiatrically "well controls."

‡ One of these two patients was optionally classifiable as either depression or alcoholism, the other as either depression or obsessive-compulsive neurosis. Each patient fulfilled criteria for both diagnoses, and it was not possible to determine that the symptoms of one disorder antedated the symptoms of the other.

‖ In all 78, including the three controls with uncomplicated mental deficiency and the four with uncomplicated epilepsy.

epilepsy. Of the remaining 32 controls with psychiatric diagnoses, seven had had their illnesses only in the past and were well at the time of the study. Thus 25 controls (23%) had current psychiatric disorders, exclusive of epilepsy or mental deficiency. In an earlier study Morrison et al.[10] collected a sample of prospective non-psychiatric controls in all age groups from the general hospital services of the same Medical Center. They found that 35% of the sample had a history of current or past psychiatric illness. That figure is comparable to the proportion of adolescent controls (N = 32, 29%) in the present study who had functional psychiatric disorders at the time of the investigation or in the past.

With respect to the types of disorders in the current study, Table 2 demonstrates that there was a predominance of typical affective syndromes and of disorders in which disturbed affect played the leading role. For example, among the 110 psychiatric inpatients, 19 had typical depression, 11 mania, 14 were called "undiagnosed, most like depression," and two were optionally classifiable between depression and another diagnosis (alcoholism in one case, obsessive-compulsive neurosis in the other case). Thus 46 (42%) of the psychiatric inpatients had an affective or predominantly affect-laden syndrome. In addition, at least some of the seven patients with a schizoaffective picture, who had an acute onset from the well state, may have had a variant of manic-depressive illness. Clayton et al.[11] have presented data from their own and other studies in support of such classification for patients suffering from this syndrome, also called "reactive schizophrenia," "remitting schizophrenia," and "schizophreniform psychosis" by various authors.[5, 12]

Only a few patients (six, 5%) received a diagnosis of schizophrenia, and one other was "undiagnosed, most like schizophrenia." This is lower than the figure cited by some other American workers who have studied adolescent inpatients. The lower figure is partly explained by the fact that in the current study the schizoaffective patients were classified separately from schizophrenics. But it is also probable that some of the manic patients and some of the "undiagnosed unclassified" group would have been diagnosed as schizophrenics at other medical centers. This issue will be discussed in Chapter 6, " 'Psychosis' and the Problem of Schizophrenia."

COMPARISION OF DIAGNOSES IN ADOLESCENTS AND IN A SAMPLE OF PSYCHIATRIC PATIENTS OF ALL AGES

To what extent did the adolescent inpatients differ from a total psychiatric inpatient group with respect to diagnostic classification? In our hospital there was no suitable "all-age" inpatient sample for comparison as to *research diagnoses* with the adolescent subjects of this study. However, with respect to *chart discharge diagnoses,* in which less strict diagnostic criteria were used, a comparison can be made between all the adolescents admitted to Renard Hospital during the study period, and all patients of any age consecutively admitted to Renard Hospital during two other periods closely adjacent in time (Table 3). In part the findings in Table 3 are explainable in terms of the incidence of various psychiatric syndromes at different times of life. For example, depression, although common among hospitalized teenagers, is even more common among hospitalized adults. By contrast, mania, schizoaffective disorders, and schizophrenia are more likely than depression to have their onsets early, and to recur or persist in adulthood. The low proportion of schizophrenics (6%) in the all-age sample is in part a reflection of the fact that these patients were in

TABLE 3

Comparison between Consecutive Admission Series of Adolescent Inpatients and Inpatients of All Ages with Respect to Chart Discharge Diagnoses

Chart Discharge Diagnoses	Psychiatric Patients of All Ages 7/15–12/31/64, 2/16–6/30/65 N = 1075	Psychiatric Patients Aged 12 to 19 9/1/65–2/27/68 N = 302
	%	%
Depression (all types)	38	26
Mania	4	4
Schizophrenia (excluding schizoaffective)	6	9
Schizoaffective	4	4
Alcoholism	13	<1
Neuroses (anxiety, hysteria, phobic, obsessional, etc.)	12	7
Personality disorders (antisocial, passive-aggressive,* sexual deviation, etc.)	5	17
Organic brain syndromes (including mental deficiency and epilepsy)	7	7
Miscellaneous (all other diagnoses, including adjustment* and stress reactions*)	2	11†
Undiagnosed*	10	15

* The fact that chart discharge diagnoses (rather than the more rigorous research diagnoses) were used for the patients in this table accounts for the relatively small proportion of undiagnosed patients. This also accounts for the use here of some terms (for example, "passive-aggressive personality" and "adolescent adjustment reaction") which have not been established as well defined syndromes by systematic studies and which were not used in the current study.

† Among adolescent patients three-quarters of the miscellaneous group were diagnosed as stress reactions or adjustment reactions.

a private, active-treatment hospital. Persons with chronic illnesses requiring long-term hospitalization are less likely to remain in an expensive facility. Patients with schizophrenia may have their earliest admissions to a private hospital, but when the chronic nature of the illness becomes clearer, families are more likely to take them to public mental hospitals for subsequent care. Alcoholism is a disorder which rarely requires hospitalization before adult life, even though heavy drinking, especially by male alcoholics, often begins in adolescence. On the other hand, proportionately more teenagers than adults are hospitalized for so-called stress reactions and adjustment reactions. This may be a reflection of a high rate of suicidal threats and behavior among young people with these diagnoses, coupled with psychiatrists' tendency to be conservative where youthful patients are concerned and to hospitalize them for lesser degrees of illness than they would adults.

Finally, in comparing hospitalized teenagers with the general psychiatric inpatient population, it is well to remind oneself that they represented only a minority, 9.7%, of the total group at Renard Hospital during the period of this investigation. Although many psychiatric disorders have their onset in youth, nevertheless, most of the disorders which fill private psychiatric hospitals, depression, alcoholism, and the various neuroses, usually do not manifest in large numbers or in more serious forms requiring hospitalization until later in life.

REFERENCES

1. Szasz, T. S. *The Myth of Mental Illness.* New York, Harper & Row, 1961.
2. Hudgens, R. W. The use of the term "undiagnosed psychiatric disorder." Br. J. Psychiatry *119:* 529–531, 1973.
3. Welner, A., Liss, J. L., Robins, E., and Richardson, M. Undiagnosed psychiatric patients: Part I: record study. Br. J. Psychiatry *120:* 315–319, 1972.
4. Stevenson, E. K., Hudgens, R. W., Held, C. P., Meredith, C. H., Hendrix, M. E., and Carr, D. L. Suicidal communication by adolescents: study of two matched groups of 60 teenagers. Dis. Nerv. Syst. *33:* 112–122, 1972.
5. Eitinger, L., Laane, C. L., and Langfeldt, C. The prognostic value of the clinical picture and the therapeutic value of physical treatment in schizophrenia and the schizophreniform states. Acta Psychiatr. Neurol. Scand. *33:* 33–53, 1958.
6. Toolan, J. M. Depression in children and adolescents. Am. J. Orthopsychiatry *32:* 404–415, 1962.
7. Offer, D. *The Psychological World of the Teenager.* New York and London, Basic Books, Inc., 1969.
8. Masterson, J. F., Jr. *The Psychiatric Dilemma of Adolescence.* Boston, Little, Brown and Co., 1967.
9. Feighner, J. P., Robins, E., Guze, S. B., Woodruff, R. A., Jr., Winokur, G., and Munoz, R. Diagnostic criteria for use in psychiatric research. Arch. Gen. Psychiatry *26:* 57–63, 1972.
10. Morrison, J. R., Hudgens, R. W., and Barchha, R. G. Life events and psychiatric illness. Br. J. Psychiatry *114:* 423–432, 1968.
11. Clayton, P. J., Rodin, L., and Winokur, G. Family history studies: III. Schizoaffective disorder, clinical and genetic factors including a one to two year follow-up. Compr. Psychiatry *9:* 31–49, 1968.
12. Vaillant, G. E. Prospective prediction of schizophrenic remission. Arch. Gen. Psychiatry *11:* 509–518, 1964.

3

Backgrounds of psychiatric inpatients and controls

MATCHING OF PSYCHIATRIC INPATIENTS AND CONTROLS

As stated in Chapter 1, the controls, who were inpatients on non-psychiatric services of the Washington University Medical Center, were selected to resemble the psychiatric inpatients as closely as possible, except with respect to a history of hospitalization (in any type of institution) for psychiatric disorder.

Table 4 compares the psychiatric patients and their controls for age, sex, race, religion, place of residence, and socioeconomic factors. The samples were similar except that significantly more of the family wage earners of psychiatric inpatients were in professional and executive occupations, and significantly more psychiatric inpatients lived in St. Louis. The latter difference was also found in a previous study of patients of all ages at the Medical Center and reflected the normal patterns of referral there.[1] Both samples had a median age of 16½ years, and two-thirds were girls. Subjects were predominantly white Protestants with private physicians in charge of their cases. Half the group came from families earning more than $10,000 a year. Only a third were from families whose wage earners were unemployed or in unskilled and semi-skilled occupations. The majority of family wage earners (usually the patients' fathers) held skilled or prestigious jobs.

In summary, the psychiatric patients and controls were matched quite well with regard to demographic factors.

MAJOR DISORDERS IN CONTROLS

The major disorders found among the controls are listed, either specifically or by general category, in Table 5. There were significant correlations between severe medical disorder and susceptibility to subsequent depression, and between antisocial personality and the occurrence of traumatic injuries. Those correlations will be discussed in the chapters dealing with those two syndromes.

TABLE 4

Comparison of Psychiatric Inpatients and Controls

	Psychiatric Patients N = 110	Controls N = 110
Age 12	5	5
13	5	5
14	9	9
15	19	18
16	11	11
17	19	19
18	18	20
19	24	23
Mean age (years)	16.50(S.D. = 2.04)	16.52(S.D. = 2.04)
Boy	44	42
Girl	66	68
White	96	98
Black	13	12
American Indian	1	0
Ever married	6	9
Protestant	76	75
Catholic	28	27
Jewish	2	7
Other	4	1
Private patients	75	84
Home in metropolitan St. Louis	57*	40*
Socioeconomic index[2] of parent ≥ 50†	47	40
Mean socioeconomic index[2] of parents†	47.8(S.D. = 26.5)	39.6(S.D. = 26.3)
Family's income above $10,000	47	55
Occupation of family's primary wage earner:		
Unemployed	9	6
Unskilled and service	11	11
Semi-skilled and operatives	15	15
Craftsmen and skilled	13	20
White collar, clerical, sales	13	14
Managers, officials, proprietors	26	30
Farmers and managers	2	6
Professional and executive	21‡	7‡

* $X^2 = 5.329$, $p < 0.05$.

† Duncan socioeconomic index[2] of father if known, of mother if father's index was unknown and mother worked. Calculated for 99 patients' parents and 109 controls' parents. The higher the score, the higher the socioeconomic level. Exceptions are 01 (unemployed) and 97 (pension, retired), which are here excluded from the calculation of mean index.

‡ X^2 corrected $= 6.916$, $p < 0.01$.

TABLE 5
Major Disorders in Controls

Principal Disorders (Including Epilepsy)	N	Psychiatric Disorders (Exclusive of Epilepsy or Mental Deficiency)				
		Definite or possible depression	Definite or possible sociopathy	Anxiety neurosis	Possible hysteria	"Undiagnosed, unclassified"
I. Traumatic injuries (recent or old)						
1. Burn, anywhere	4	2	1			
2. Gunshot, anywhere	2		1			
3. Facial injury, not burn or gun	11	1	2			
4. Injury to limb, not burn or gun	9		1			
5. Head injury, not burn or gun	1					
II. Non-traumatic, surgical						
1. Elective plastic surgery	15	1				
2. Congenital heart disease	4	1				
3. Appendicitis	4	2				
4. Miscellaneous*	11	1		1	1	1
III. Nonsurgical treatment						
1. Malignancy, disseminated	6	4				
2. Epilepsy	6	1	1			
3. Severe renal	4					
4. Diabetes mellitus	4					
5. Lupus erythematosus	3	1				
6. Hepatitis	3					
7. Obesity	3	1				1
8. Asthma	2	1				
9. Rheumatoid arthritis	2	1				
10. Neuromuscular, structural change	2	1				
11. Pain, no structural change	4	2				
12. Infection, not listed above	5					
13. Miscellaneous, structural change†	5	2				

* Inguinal hernia; ganglion cyst; colon cyst; cholelithiasis; hyperplasia of cervix; cervical ribs; hypospadias; scoliosis; testicular infarction; ureteral obstruction; intestinal adhesions.

† Erythema nodosum; iron deficiency anemia; bronchiectasis; ulcerative colitis; rickets.

COMPARISONS AMONG PSYCHIATRIC INPATIENTS, PSYCHIATRICALLY ILL CONTROLS AND PSYCHIATRICALLY WELL CONTROLS

A substantial number of controls had psychiatric illnesses, currently or in the past, as defined by the presence of disability from disturbed thinking, mood, or behavior, even though adolescents with a history of prior psychiatric *hospitalization* were excluded from consideration as controls (see Chapter 2). In the course of this chapter, the 110 psychiatric inpatients will be compared with two subgroups of the control sample: those who never had a psychiatric disorder, and those who had. In this way it may be ascertained in what ways, if any, these three groups differed with respect to medical, sociologic, and emotional factors, and various features of life history. It is recognized that the value of comparisons among these three samples is limited to some extent because of the heterogeneity within each sample with respect to diagnoses and the degrees of severity of illnesses. The significance of these latter factors will be explored in this and subsequent chapters.

The psychiatrically ill controls were the 32 general hospital patients who had psychiatric disorders either at the time of the study (25 patients) or in the past (seven patients). This group included two youths with epilepsy who were scored as psychiatrically ill because one had an antisocial personality and the other an undiagnosed illness "most like depression." These 32 patients will be referred to hereafter as "sick" or "ill" controls.

The remaining 78 non-psychiatric inpatients were the psychiatrically well controls. Four of them had epilepsy, and three had mental deficiency without apparent emotional impairment. Their cases were psychiatrically uncomplicated. These 78 subjects will be termed "well controls" in this chapter, though of course they did have non-psychiatric disorders.

Demographic Characteristics

The three groups, 110 psychiatric inpatients, 32 psychiatrically ill controls, and 78 psychiatrically well controls were similar with respect to sex distribution, race, and marital status. The sick controls were slightly older (mean 17.0 years, S.D. 2.0) than the well controls (16.3 years, S.D. 2.0). This difference was not quite significant (t-test of pooled variance 1.67, $p > 0.05$) and might in part be explained because older controls were at risk for psychiatric disorders for a longer period of time.

The psychiatric inpatients resembled the ill controls and differed from the well controls with regard to the proportion living in Metropolitan St. Louis ($X^2 = 8.2$, $p < 0.01$), and proportion in staff (non-private) care ($X^2 = 4.8$, $p < 0.05$). Thus the adolescents with psychiatric illness, whether they were psychiatric inpatients or controls on the medical services, were more likely to be city dwellers and ward-care patients. However, the families of sick controls and well controls were similar regarding mean Duncan socioeconomic index[2] (39.5 and 39.2, respectively), the proportion having a socioeconomic index of at least 50 (38.7% and 38.5%), and the proportion earning $10,000 or more in the preceding year (50.1% and

51.3%). Over-all, the demographic similarities among the three comparison groups were impressive and the differences less so.

Psychiatric Disorders among Subjects' Parents

There was a significantly higher incidence of a history of psychiatric disorders and deviant behavior among parents of psychiatrically ill adolescents (both the psychiatric inpatients and the sick controls), than among parents of well controls (Table 6). This finding has been common in other studies. The data in Table 6 were systematically collected from the 220 adolescents and from 209 of the parents themselves. Thus much of the information about parents was gathered first-hand from the subjects of the inquiry and was supplemented by direct observations of the parents by the interviewers.

Even though psychiatric illness was less severe among the 32 ill controls than among the 110 psychiatric inpatients, those two groups did not differ significantly as to the proportion with parents who had been jailed, nonsupporting, heavy drinkers, or psychiatrically ill. This suggests that psychiatric disorders in the parents of sick controls might have operated as causative factors of psychiatric illness in the children through biologic or environmental influences, or both.

Inspection of Table 6 shows that, as far as the three specified forms of deviant behavior were concerned, heavy drinking was something of a common denominator. For example, 29% of the psychiatric inpatients had

TABLE 6

*History of Deviant Behavior and Psychiatric Illness in Parents**

	Psychiatric Inpatients N = 110	Ill Controls N = 32	Well Controls N = 78
	%	%	%
At least one parent† jailed	9	19	3
At least one parent† not steady worker or productive	11	6	1
At least one parent† heavy drinker	25	22	10
At least one parent in one of above categories	29	28	13
Psychiatric illness in natural mother	24	38	8
Psychiatric illness in natural father	30	28	14
Psychiatric illness in both natural parents (includes totals above)	8	13	0
Psychiatric illness in at least one natural parent	46	53	22

* Differences between psychiatrically ill subjects (inpatients and controls) and well controls were significant for all items: highest $p < 0.01$.

† Step or adoptive parents are here listed among those jailed, drinking heavily, or not working steadily only if they lived with subject at the time of the deviant behavior. Otherwise only natural parents are listed.

at least one parent who was either jailed, drank heavily, or did not work steadily, and 25% had a parent who drank heavily. Thus 86% of the behavioral deviation occurred in parents who drank heavily.

In all, 97 of the subjects' 440 natural parents, 53 fathers and 44 mothers, were known to have had disability from disorders of thought, mood, or behavior (22%). Among fathers, there were 37 with alcoholism, nine with depression, two with antisocial personality, and five with disorders of an undetermined type. Unipolar depression, as distinct from manic-depressive (bipolar) illness, was the leading disorder among mothers, 21 of whom had this syndrome, whereas only three were alcoholics or drug abusers. Three mothers had hysteria, two schizophrenia, one bipolar manic-depressive illness, one anxiety neurosis, one mental deficiency, and 12 an undetermined type of illness. Some of the 12 mothers and five fathers with undetermined types of disorders may have had schizophrenia, affective disorder, anxiety neurosis, or hysteria. Since research methods did not include a symptom survey for the parents or a search of parents' psychiatric records, and since many of the parents were sick only in the past, some of their disorders could not be definitely diagnosed by the investigators at the time of this study. Thus alcoholism and affective disorders were by far the most common parental illnesses, accounting for at least 73% of the cases. There was a predominance of depression in the mothers and alcoholism in the fathers.

The finding of so many depressed parents is not surprising in view of the high incidence of affective illnesses among the psychiatrically ill adolescents. The high proportion of alcoholic fathers, both among adolescents with affective disorder and those with antisocial traits is in keeping with the findings of Winokur and associates[3] that alcoholism appears with unexpected frequency among male relatives of unipolar depressives, and the findings of Robins[4] that alcoholism is prevalent among the fathers of sociopaths. Our figures also suggest that alcoholism may be the eventual fate of some of our study subjects who were as yet too young to have fully developed the syndrome. As will be discussed later in this chapter, some of our adolescents had drinking habits which suggested that they might be on their way to alcoholism, whereas two were already definite alcoholics.

Psychiatric Disorders among Siblings

Few of the subjects' 652 siblings had lived very long in the ages of risk for common psychiatric disorders. Accordingly, figures of incidence would not be meaningful. Eighteen percent of psychiatric inpatients, 6% of ill controls, and 8% of well controls, had at least one psychiatrically ill sibling. Since the siblings were rarely interviewed, it was seldom possible to make diagnoses with confidence.

Psychiatric Disorders among Remote Relatives

At least one psychiatrically ill remote relative (grandparent, uncle, aunt, cousin) was reported for 65% of the psychiatric inpatients, 44% of the ill controls, and 40% of the well controls. Insofar as diagnoses could be conjectured for this group, alcoholism and depression seemed by far the most prevalent disorders. Of 115 subjects for whom psychiatrically ill remote relatives were reported, there were 52 (45%) with at least one depressed remote relative and 37 (32%) with at least one alcoholic remote relative. There were 34 additional subjects who had sick remote relatives whose type of illness could not be identified. Because of the large number of remote relatives and their varying degrees of consanguinity with our subjects and because remote relatives were not interviewed directly, we did not try to obtain data about the actual incidence of various disorders in the group.

Severity of Psychiatric Disorders among Relatives

There were two indices of severity of psychiatric disorder in patients' relatives, hospitalization and suicide. There were no significant differences among the three comparison groups with respect to the proportion for whom hospitalization of remote relatives was reported. But psychiatric hospitalization of at least one primary relative was reported for 24% of psychiatric inpatients, 13% of psychiatrically ill controls, and 7% of psychiatrically well controls. The difference between the combined psychiatrically ill groups and the well controls was significant (X^2 corrected 6.88, $p < 0.01$). Only one primary relative of a subject had committed suicide, the alcoholic father of a psychiatric inpatient. Suicide was reported among remote relatives by 12% of psychiatric inpatients, 9% of sick controls, and 8% of well controls.

In summary, the relatives of the study subjects who were psychiatrically ill showed a prevalence of affective disorders and alcoholism. Differences in incidence and severity of psychiatric disorders among the three adolescent comparison groups—psychiatric inpatients, sick controls, and well controls—were most significant with respect to the parents (the only first-degree relatives who had lived well into the ages of risk for psychiatric illnesses). For the remote relatives, differences among the groups were less impressive.

Separation from Parents, Bereavement, and Parental Divorce

Table 7 summarizes major separation and bereavement experiences during the lifetimes of the subjects. There were no intergroup differences significant at the 0.05 level, even when the two psychiatrically ill samples

TABLE 7

*Separation and Bereavement Experiences**

	Psychiatric Inpatients N = 110	Ill Controls N = 32	Well Controls N = 78
	%	%	%
Death of a parent	13	6	6
Death of a sibling	5	9	1
Divorce of parents or separation of more than one year	19	22	23
Separation of subject from one parent for more than two months other than for above reasons	13	10	8
Separation of subject from both parents for more than two months other than for above reasons	35	29	26

* No significant differences between groups for any item.

were compared with the well controls, but the data merit detailed examination.

Parents' Death

In the total group of 220 subjects, 21 parental deaths were reported: 16 natural fathers, three natural mothers, one adoptive father, and one stepfather. It is of interest that five of the 21 deaths were ascribable to the complications of psychiatric illness. The illness was alcoholism in all five cases, and all the decedents were natural parents of psychiatrically ill subjects. One father and one mother died of cirrhosis, two fathers were killed in automobile accidents while intoxicated, and one father committed suicide. The deaths occurred from one to 12 years before the study admissions of the subjects.

Of the remaining 16 parental deaths, 14 were natural, two violent. Both the latter were parents of psychiatric patients: the mother of one was killed in an accident, and the stepfather of another was killed by the patient herself. The latter parent, although not scored as psychiatrically ill and not a heavy drinker, had an erratic and violent temper and habitually beat and verbally abused his stepdaughter for years until she shot him to death when she was 15 years old.

Thus all five parental deaths which were ascribable to psychiatric illness, and both the other violent deaths, occurred in the families of psychiatric inpatients or psychiatrically ill controls. The number of parental deaths was too small to draw conclusions about whether there were critical ages at which a child was more likely to be made susceptible to psychiatric disorder because of a parent's death. However, we found an unexpectedly high incidence of paternal deaths among subjects with antisocial traits (see Chapters 7 and 8). In fact, three of the six sociopaths who lost their fathers began significant antisocial behavior immediately after the bereavement.

Siblings' Deaths

Few subjects had siblings who died, and there were no significant differences among psychiatric inpatients, well controls, and ill controls. Seven subjects had lost one sibling, and two had lost two siblings. Five of these 11 siblings died at birth and four others were two years or younger. One 18-year-old brother (not psychiatrically ill) died in an automobile accident, and one 36-year-old half brother died of alcoholic cirrhosis. The last was the sibling of a psychiatric inpatient who was "undiagnosed, most like sociopathy."

Separation from Parents and Parental Divorce

It is surprising that divorce and long term separation of parents were no more common among psychiatrically ill subjects than among the well controls,* in view of findings in other studies and in view of the higher incidence of psychiatric problems among parents of psychiatrically ill patients in this investigation. But this finding emphasizes once again the sociologic similarity between the psychiatric patients and the control groups in the present study. The three groups did not differ significantly as to the age of the patients at the time of their parents' separations or divorces.

The three comparison groups also did not differ with respect to incidence of periods of two months or longer living apart from parents when separations caused by death, divorce, or parents' long term martial separations were excluded. This remained true whether all separation experiences were considered, or whether the *patients'* leaving the home for any reason (school, military service, hospitalization) was considered apart from one or both *parents* leaving the home.

Table 8 compares the three groups with regard to a quantitative factor in the bereavement-separation experiences, the length of time the subjects lived with only one parent (natural, step, or adoptive) due to parental divorce or separation or parental death. Once again the similarity among the groups is demonstrated.

In summary, as a total group the psychiatric inpatients and ill controls did not differ significantly from the well controls with respect to the incidence or separation or bereavement experiences. However, parental deaths and marital disruption may have had a significant effect on the

* The "undiagnosed, unclassified" subsample had a higher incidence of parental divorce. This will be discussed in Chapter 8.

TABLE 8

*Cumulative Time Subjects Lived with Only One Parent**

	Psychiatric Inpatients N = 110	Ill Controls N = 32	Well Controls N = 78
	%	%	%
Due to separation or divorce of parents			
Not applicable	80	78	76
Some time, but unknown	0	3	6
Less than six months	4	0	3
Six months, less than one year	5	6	1
One to five years	5	6	6
More than five years	7	6	8
Due to death of parent			
Not applicable	87	94	94
Less than six months	1	0	1
Six months, less than one year	5	0	0
One to five years	6	6	1
More than five years	1	0	4

* No significant differences between groups for any item.

TABLE 9

Number of Siblings and Birth Order

	Psychiatric Inpatients N = 110	Ill Controls N = 32	Well Controls N = 78
	%	%	%
Number siblings (natural, step, or adoptive) in home of rearing when subject was between ages 5 and 15:*			
None	12	13	5
One	22	16	15
Two	17	22	28
Three	20	3	17
Four	9	28	13
Five	11	13	6
More than five	9	6	15
Birth order:			
Subject only child	12	13	5
Oldest of sibship	30	31	35
Youngest of sibship	25	16	15
Neither oldest nor youngest	34	41	45
Mean number of siblings	2.73(S.D. = 2.07)	3.13(S.D. = 2.6)	3.29(S.D. = 2.50)

* The only significant difference between groups was that the well controls were more likely than the psychiatric inpatients to have more than one sibling: $X^2 = 3.88$, $p < 0.05$.

sociopathic behavior and emotional instability of some of the teenagers with antisocial personality and an "undiagnosed, unclassified" syndrome. These issues will be discussed in Chapters 7 and 8.

Composition of the Homes

Tables 9, 10, and 11 deal with the birth order of the subjects, number of siblings in the homes of rearing, the identity of the current functional parents, and living arrangements at the time of the study. Differences among the three groups with respect to any of these factors were unimpressive. On the contrary, the data tabulated here underscore the similarity among the comparison groups as to the composition of their homes in the past and currently.

TABLE 10

*Current Family Configurations**

	Psychiatric Inpatients N = 110	Ill Controls N = 32	Well Controls N = 78
	%	%	%
Natural parents are the functional parents	70	69	68
Natural mother, substitute father	8	13	12
Natural father, substitute mother	1	0	0
Substitute father and mother	5	0	3
Natural father, no current mother	0	6	0
Substitute father, no current mother	0	0	0
Natural mother, no current father	12	13	15
Substitute mother, no current father	4	0	3
No current functional parents	1	0	0

* No significant differences between groups.

TABLE 11

*Current Living Arrangements**

	Psychiatric Inpatients N = 110	Ill Controls N = 32	Well Controls N = 78
	%	%	%
Lives with two parents (one or both may be natural, step, or adoptive)	81	69	77
Lives with only one parent	12	16	17
Lives with spouse	5	9	5
Lives with friend of opposite sex	0	3	0
Lives in an institution or in Job Corps	2	3	1

* No significant differences between groups.

Attitudes of Subjects toward Parents

Each subject was asked the open-ended questions: "Tell me about your parents (step or foster parents if they were the current functional parents). What are (or were) they like? How have you gotten along with them?" The responses were scored as to whether they expressed predominantly positive, negative, mixed, or neutral (bland) attitudes. The results are summarized in Table 12. These data reflect the subjective impressions of the adolescents, not objective or systematic observation by the investigators of parent-child interaction. Since the teenagers were interviewed at the time of hospitalization, their impressions were colored by their illnesses, and by the often conflictful events preceding hospital admission for psychiatric problems. It has been shown (for example, by Murphy *et al.*,[5] and Morrison *et al.*[1]) that psychiatric disorders are accompanied by more conflict between patients and relatives than non-psychiatric disorders. Therefore, the data in Table 12, which show considerably more negative attitudes toward parents by psychiatrically ill adolescents, cannot be demonstrated to have etiologic significance for psychiatric disorders; although, of course, long standing interpersonal conflicts could conceivably have contributed to the incidence and mode of expression of psychiatric disorder and perhaps to the crises leading to hospital admission of the psychiatrically ill group. The reverse, however, is certainly true: the symptoms of psychiatric disorders in the teenage subjects, especially the

TABLE 12

Attitudes to Parents Expressed by Subjects

	Psychiatric Inpatients N = 110	Ill Controls N = 32	Well Controls N = 78
	%	%	%
Neutral or bland attitude to both parents	9	3	0
Positive to both parents*	30	53	77
Positive, has only one functional parent	1	0	1
Positive to mother, negative to father	18	6	10
Positive to father, negative to mother	4	3	3
Mixed to both parents	19	9	6
Negative to both parents†	13	16	1
Negative, has only one functional parent	2	6	0
No response	4	3	1
Unclassifiable response	1	0	0

* Significantly fewer psychiatric inpatients reported positive attitudes toward both parents than did sick controls ($p < 0.01$) or well controls ($p < 0.001$), and fewer sick controls than well controls reported such attitudes ($p < 0.05$).

† Significantly more psychiatrically ill subjects (psychiatric inpatients and sick controls combined) reported negative attitudes to both parents than did the psychiatrically well controls, $p < 0.01$.

irritability and deviant behavior of the sociopaths, contributed to a deterioration of relationships among the subjects and their parents.

Medical Histories

Prenatal and Perinatal Disorders

Of the 102 psychiatric inpatients for whom such information was known, only eight (8%) were not born in a hospital. This was true of 6% of 31 psychiatrically ill controls and 3% of 76 well controls. The same insignificant differences were found among the three groups with respect to complications during pregnancy of the subjects' mothers: 8% of 100 psychiatric patients, 6% of 32 sick controls, 3% of 76 well controls. Of the 12 mothers in all groups reporting complications while they were pregnant with the subjects, ten had non-traumatic disorders (for example, infections), one a traumatic injury, one a psychiatric illness (this was the mother of a psychiatric inpatient).

Perinatal medical problems—prematurity, cyanosis, breach birth, cesarean delivery, injuries, illnesses, etc.—were reported for 9% of 101 psychiatric patients, 3% of the 32 sick controls, and 8% of 76 well controls. None of these differences were significant at the 5% level. Of the 209 subjects for whom such information was known, the most frequent complication, prematurity (which was specifically inquired about), was reported for only 4%. This was defined as a statement by the parent or on the hospital maternity record that the subject was premature or that he weighed under five pounds at birth.

Injuries and Illness

Table 13 compares the three groups for histories of traumatic injuries and non-traumatic illnesses at any time in life after the perinatal period. The hospitalization record (last item in Table 13) here includes psychiatric hospitalization as well. This table is a general measure of ill health—medical, surgical, and psychiatric—over the subjects' entire lifetimes. The groups were strikingly similar in this respect. The only item in the table that significantly differentiated the groups was "injuries to more than one part of the body." None such traumata were reported for the well controls, which was thus significantly less than for the psychiatric patients (<0.05) and psychiatrically ill controls (<0.01). Data will be presented in Chapter 7 demonstrating an association between antisocial personality and traumatic injuries in the ill controls.

One item related to growth and development, and not tabulated with the illnesses, differentiated psychiatric inpatients and the psychiatrically ill controls. Twenty-three of 60 girls (38%) in the former group and 14 of 20 (70%) in the latter group had not menstruated by their 13th birthday

TABLE 13

*Illnesses and Injuries during Subjects' Lifetimes after Perinatal Period**

	Psychiatric Inpatients N = 110	Ill Controls N = 32	Well Controls N = 78
	%	%	%
Traumatic injuries†			
Injuries to limbs	20	19	14
Injuries to head	28	22	19
Injuries to trunk	8	9	3
Injuries to more than one body area (also scored above)	7	13	0
No injuries or only minor lacerations, slight sprains, etc.	53	63	64
Non-traumatic Illnesses			
Only common childhood viral disorders, no hospitalization (colds, measles, etc.)	16	16	18
Other type non-traumatic disorders, no hospitalization (rheumatic fever, bronchitis, pneumonia, allergies)	4	3	1
Combination of viral and other type disorders, no hospitalization	3	0	4
Non-traumatic disorders of any type (including psychiatric) requiring prior hospitalization	77	81	78

* All injuries are listed, including those leading to admission, but the current episode of *non-traumatic* illness is not listed here for controls.

† Percentages for injuries total more than 100% because of multiple injuries in some patients.

($p < 0.05$). Such a significant difference was not noted among the other group comparisons and may be related to the fact that the psychiatrically ill controls were the most medically ill of the three comparison groups, hence perhaps more likely to have a delayed sexual maturation.

Nonpsychiatric Hospitalization

The data in Table 14 concern prior hospitalization for non-psychiatric disorders. Here some differences among the three groups emerge, because the controls were selected from a medically ill population, and could be expected to have more serious disorders of those types in their backgrounds. Inspection of the table reveals that the psychiatric inpatients had a history of being more healthy (medically) than the psychiatrically well controls, who in turn had been more healthy than the psychiatrically ill controls. Eighty-one percent of the ill controls had previously been in a non-psychiatric hospital, compared to 76% of well controls and 64% of the psychiatric inpatients. These differences between

TABLE 14

Prior Hospitalization for Non-psychiatric Disorders

	Psychiatric Inpatients N = 110	Ill Controls N = 32	Well Controls N = 78
	%	%	%
Number prior hospitalizations, lifetime			
Never hospitalized before	36	19	24
Hospitalized once	33	9	22
Hospitalized twice	14	22	23
Hospitalized three times*	8	16	9
More than three times*	9	34	22
Cumulative prior time in hospitals, lifetime			
None	36	19	24
Some, duration unknown	4	9	15
Less than two weeks	35	22	35
Two weeks to one month†	7	19	12
More than one month†	8	31	14

* Ill controls were more likely than psychiatric inpatients to have been hospitalized more than twice or more than three times ($p < 0.01$). This was also true when well controls were compared with psychiatric inpatients ($p < 0.05$).

† Significantly more of the ill controls than of the psychiatric inpatients ($p < 0.001$) or than of the well controls ($p < 0.02$) had more than two weeks of prior hospitalization. Significantly more ill controls than psychiatric inpatients had been hospitalized more than one month ($p < 0.05$).

groups were not striking, but significant differences are evident when one takes into account the number of prior hospitalizations and the cumulative time in hospitals. Compared to psychiatric inpatients, the ill controls and well controls were more likely to have been hospitalized more than twice or more than three times. With respect to amount of time previously spent in non-psychiatric hospitals, the psychiatric inpatients resembled the psychiatrically well controls, whereas the psychiatrically ill controls had more prior hospital time than either of the other groups. Of ill controls, 50% had more than two weeks prior hospitalization, compared to 15% of psychiatric inpatients ($p < 0.001$) and 22% of well controls ($p < 0.02$). The ill controls also differed significantly from the psychiatric inpatients with respect to proportions hospitalized more than one month. Even among the psychiatrically ill controls, however, only 16% had spent an accumulation of more than three months in hospitals, and none had been in for more than a year. On the whole, the subjects of the study were acutely, not chronically, ill.

In summary, the three comparison groups were generally alike with respect to the amount of ill health during their lives. However, there was a tendency for psychiatrically ill controls to have a history of more serious non-psychiatric disorders than psychiatrically well controls or psychiatric inpatients. It will be shown in Chapter 4 that the presence of severe medical disorders in controls may have played a role in the precipitation of depressive syndromes.

Intelligence Quotients Measured in Schools

The three comparison groups were similar with respect to intelligence. I.Q.'s were available from the school records of 90 of the 110 psychiatric inpatients, 26 of the 28 sick controls, and 61 of the 78 well controls. A variety of tests had been used, most often the California, Otis, and Kuhlman. Among the psychiatric inpatients, the highest I.Q. recorded was under 100 for 20% of psychiatric inpatients, 23% of sick controls, and 16% of well controls. It was above 120 for 27% of psychiatric inpatients, 19% of sick controls, and 38% of well controls. These differences among the groups were not statistically significant. With respect to the mean I.Q.'s, the three groups were almost identical: 112 (S.D. = 16.7) for psychiatric inpatients, 110 (S.D. = 14.6) for sick controls, and 112 (S.D. = 16.7) for well controls.

There were 22 psychiatric inpatients, 11 sick controls, and 11 well controls who had been retested with the same I.Q. test three or more years after it had been first administered. An additional 29 psychiatric inpatients, 6 sick controls, and 14 well controls had been administered different tests after at least a three-year interval. Thus 54% of the subjects for whom we had I.Q. data had been retested at least once. As shown in Table 15, comparable proportions of the three groups showed changes in I.Q. scores over time. The differences among the samples did not approach significance for any of the comparisons.

TABLE 15

*I.Q. Score Changes over at Least a Three-Year Interval**

	Retest More than 10 Points below Original	Retest More than 10 Points above Original
	%	%
Same test		
Psychiatric inpatients (N = 22)	23	14
Psychiatrically ill controls (N = 11)	18	27
Psychiatrically well controls (N = 11)	27	9
Different test only		
Psychiatric inpatients (N = 29)	24	31
Psychiatrically ill controls (N = 6)	0	17
Psychiatrically well controls (N = 14)	28	14

* No differences between groups at <5% level of significance.

Interest and Activities

Not only were the three subject groups of comparable intelligence, they had comparable interests as well. Each subject was asked, in an open-ended question, to discuss his major interests and activities in school and outside school. Replies were spontaneous: the different areas were not systematically inquired about.

As a group the adolescent subjects of this investigation expressed spontaneous interest in both school work and extracurricular activities. Athletics and liberal arts were most popular, religion the least popular of the categories. Only a small minority failed to express active interest or to demonstrate involvement in activities.

Table 16 demonstrates the similarities among the groups in their interests. Only one of 39 intergroup comparisons showed a significant difference between groups. One such finding was to be expected among such a large number of comparisons, and no real importance can be attached to it.

Sexual History

Approximately the same proportion of subjects in each comparison sample had dated members of the opposite sex by the time of the study—

TABLE 16

*Spontaneously Expressed Interests and Participation in Activities**

	Psychiatric Inpatients N = 110	Ill Controls N = 32	Well Controls N = 78%
	%	%	%
Related to school			
Science, mathematics	38	38	41
Liberal arts	55	41	58
Fine arts	25†	13	10†
No interest expressed	11	9	4
Only active disinterest	5	3	3
Not related to school			
Social	44	53	50
Athletics	57	59	68
Religious	8	9	6
Fine arts	25	22	27
Nonartistic technical	29	28	19
Liberal arts	18	6	10
No interest expressed	5	6	1
Only active disinterest	6	0	3

* Totals exceeded 100% because of multiple interests expressed.

† X^2 corrected = 5.9, $p < 0.02$.

71% of psychiatric inpatients, 78% of sick controls, and 73% of well controls. The groups began dating at approximately the same mean ages—14.3, 14.6, and 14.8 years, respectively. At the time of the study, among those subjects who were at least 15 years old (N = 182), 8% were married, and 39% of the single adolescents were dating at least once a week. There were very small differences among the three comparison groups with respect to these factors.

Although similar proportions of the three comparison groups had dated, and although they began dating at about the same mean ages, the groups differed significantly with respect to reported sexual experience. Thirty-nine percent of the psychiatric inpatients, 47% of the psychiatrically ill controls, and only 17% of the psychiatrically well controls said they had had intercourse with a member of the opposite sex. The differences between the well controls and each of the two psychiatrically ill groups was significant at <0.01. The well controls who had intercourse first did so at a later mean age, 16.6 years, than did the psychiatric inpatients (15.4) or the psychiatrically ill controls (15.8). Furthermore, among those subjects who were at least 17 years old and who had had intercourse, intimacy with more than one partner was reported by 21 of 33 psychiatric inpatients (64%), eight of 13 sick controls (62%) and only three of 11 well controls (27%). Intercourse with five or more partners was reported, respectively, by 36%, 23%, and 9% of those subject groups.

Homosexual relationships were reported only by the psychiatric inpatients, 10% of whom told of such experiences. None of the controls reported this.

The higher proportion of psychiatrically ill adolescents with a history of sexual experience was a reflection of the generally venturesome behavior of those patients with antisocial character traits. The subject will be discussed in Chapter 7.

Scholastic Performance and Behavior in School

The three subject groups, with their generally comparable levels of intelligence, entered school at comparable ages. Of 109 psychiatric inpatients, 92 entered first grade before their seventh birthday, all before their eighth. Only 4 of the 109 controls (psychiatrically ill or well) entered school after they were seven years old.

Table 17 gives a general estimate of academic problems and of behavioral problems in school. Here the psychiatrically well controls fared best, the psychiatric inpatients not as well, and the psychiatrically ill controls worst. The well controls had a significantly lower incidence of trouble in every category compared to the other two groups when the latter were combined. As will be seen later, school problems were most frequently found in youths with antisocial personality. But this syndrome

TABLE 17

*School Problems over Lifetimes of Subjects**

	Psychiatric Inpatients N = 110	Ill Controls N = 32	Well Controls N = 78
	%	%	%
Suspension or expulsion for misbehavior	21	16	4
Truant more than once a year	23	31	12
In trouble for fighting	14	16	6
Held back at least one semester, academic reasons	18	19	10
Discontinued school (out at least one semester at time of study admission)	21	37	13
Trouble in at least one of the above categories	52	72	28

* In all categories the combined groups of psychiatric inpatients and psychiatrically ill controls had a significantly higher proportion for whom problems were reported than did the well control group.

did not account for the high incidence of trouble in the psychiatrically ill adolescents of this study, since only 14 of 110 psychiatric inpatients and six of 110 controls had definite or possible antisocial personality. Psychiatric illness in general has a disruptive influence on school performance.

Getting in trouble for fighting in school was a characteristic of the preteen years. This behavior was reported for 25 subjects and had begun and ended by 8th grade in 19 (76%). The only subjects for whom any trouble with fighting was reported in high school were those who first began fighting in high school. In general, trouble with fighting did not continue for very long. It was reported to have extended over more than two years in only three of 25 subjects.

Thirty-nine of the 220 subjects had been held back in school for academic reasons: four for one semester, 15 for two semesters (one school year), and the remainder for three to five semesters. This, like trouble with fighting, was a feature of the earlier years in school, happening after sixth grade in only nine of 39 subjects.

Truancy occurred in 44 of the 220 subjects and was predominantly a high school phenomenon, beginning for the first time after the 8th grade in 64% of those truanting. In those who began truancy earlier, it ended earlier: 12 of the 15 subjects who had first been truant before high school had stopped this behavior before high school began.

Of the 31 subjects in all groups who had ever been expelled or suspended for misbehavior, 20 had been expelled only once, seven expelled two or three times, and four more than three times. Eighteen of the 31 subjects who were expelled or suspended had first experienced this difficulty in high school. On the other hand, if expulsion or suspension was reported to have occurred for the first time before the ninth grade (13 subjects), it usually had terminated before ninth grade (11 subjects).

Of the 44 subjects who had been out of school at least one semester at the time of our study, 18 had left school at a normal termination point (one after eighth grade, 17 upon graduation from high school). The remaining 26 had dropped out, either before eighth grade (3), during high school (16) or college (7).

In summary, the pattern of school trouble, when it occurred, was for fighting and grade repeating to begin early, in elementary school or junior high, and for truancy and expulsion to begin in high school. With respect to each type of problem, there was a tendency for the troubles which began early to terminate before high school. By contrast, troubles which were reported to have occurred at all in high school were likely to have begun in those years.

Employment

Among the 110 psychiatric inpatients, 49% had had some kind of job, as compared with 41% of the psychiatrically sick controls and only 22% of the well controls, a significantly lower figure (Table 18). This may have been related in part to the fact that a higher proportion of the psychiatrically ill adolescents had stopped going to school. Of the 54 psychiatric inpatients who had ever held jobs, 12 (22%) had had personal difficulties on the job and three had been discharged once because of the problems. None of the 13 sick controls reported such problems, but three of the 17 well controls who had worked reported personal problems and all three had been discharged once (18%). Job impairment because of psychiatric symptoms was reported for 13 (24%) of the 54 psychiatric inpatients who had worked, one of the 13 working sick controls, and none of

TABLE 18

*Jobs Held by Subjects**

	Psychiatric Inpatients N = 110	Ill Controls N = 32	Well Controls N = 78
	%	%	%
No job ever†	51	59	78
Vacation jobs	28	13	14
Regular job concurrent with school	24	9	5
Regular job or military service while not enrolled in school	15	25	6

* Proportions total more than 100% because some subjects held jobs in more than one category.

† Psychiatrically ill subjects (inpatients and controls) had held jobs more often than well controls, $p < 0.01$.

the well controls. Medical problems had impaired the work of two psychiatric inpatients (2%), five sick controls (38%), and 4 well controls (23%). These findings of course correlate with the greater severity of psychiatric problems among the psychiatric inpatients and of medical problems in both control groups, whether psychiatrically sick or psychiatrically well.

Arrests

Deviant behavior, as might be expected, was significantly more frequent among the psychiatrically ill adolescents in both the psychiatric inpatient and sick control groups than among the well controls. There was a history of arrests for 14% of the 110 psychiatric inpatients, 25% of the sick controls, and only 4% of the well controls. The intergroup comparisons between each psychiatrically ill group and the well group were significant at <0.05. Of the 26 subjects in the total study sample who had ever been arrested, one had been arrested only for traffic offenses and less than four times for those. Ten had been arrested for misconduct or for four or more traffic offenses, 10 for crimes against property, one for crimes against persons, and four both for misconduct and crimes against property.

Those arrested among the psychiatric inpatients had a mean of 2.7 arrests, with six of the 15 reporting more than three arrests. For the psychiatrically ill controls there were a mean of 1.5 arrests, with none arrested more than three times. All three of the well controls who had been arrested reported having this experience only once. Nine of the 16 arrested psychiatric inpatients had been in prison or detention, compared to none of the sick controls and one well control. Thus, although a smaller proportion of psychiatric inpatients than sick controls had been arrested, those arrested in the former group had had more arrests and had been in more serious trouble for their deviant behavior.

The mean age for first arrest was 15.2 years for the total arrested sample in all three groups, with no arrests before age 12 and with 43% of the sample first arrested at age 16 or older.

Use of Alcohol and Drugs

Systematic inquiry was made of all subjects and parents about the use of alcohol and of all drugs, whether or not they were prescribed by physicians and whether they were obtained through legal or illegal channels. Ten questions concerned the use of drugs and 24 the use of alcohol, with attention to social, medical, and psychiatric effects of all substances. This section of the chapter is concerned with the use of alcohol, which is technically illegal for persons under 21 in Missouri, and the use of *non-*

prescribed drugs, both standard agents which are prescribed under other circumstances (for example, barbiturates and amphetamines) and illegal agents (*e.g.,* marijuana, LSD, and heroin).

In this study the inappropriate use of drugs and the abuse of alcohol were confined almost exclusively to the psychiatric inpatients, and drinking was definitely more prevalent than drug use among those psychiatrically ill teenagers at the time of the investigation, 1965 to 1968. It is the clinical impression of the author that the use of the drugs inquired about may have increased among white middle class teenagers in the St. Louis area since that time. Non-systematic surveys in suburban high schools and conversations with psychiatrically well teenagers in 1970 and 1971 have indicated that there is experimental or occasional use of marijuana, for example, by at least one-third to one-half the student bodies in such schools. Similar clinical impressions also suggest that there is still a very low incidence of marijuana or psychedelic drug use among teenagers in the rural areas of Missouri and Illinois.

In any case, the investigators in the current study distinguished between moderate use of drugs or alcohol and abuse of these substances among our subjects. It is of interest that drug abuse did not play a leading role in the manifestations of psychiatric disorders among many of these teenagers, in spite of the fact that they were sick enough to be hospitalized. Even though drug use among St. Louis area youths may have increased since 1968, nevertheless drugs were a popular subject of conversation among teenagers and of concern by their parents even then. Among the subjects of this study, at least, the psychopathology that preceded or led to drug and alcohol abuse seemed far more important than the abuse of the substances themselves.

Sixty-six (60%) of the 110 psychiatric inpatients, 50% of the 32 psychiatrically ill controls, and 26% of the 78 psychiatrically well controls had a history of some alcohol consumption. This was mild and problem-free behavior among all the well controls, and among all but one of the psychiatrically ill controls. By contrast, nine of the psychiatric inpatients had a history of regular drinking that was excessive currently (seven patients) or in the past (two patients), according to the patients themselves or their families. Four other inpatients had a history of drinking amounts of alcohol that were socially inappropriate for age (*e.g.,* 12 years) or circumstances.

In 20 of the psychiatric inpatients, even among some who had not been heavy drinkers, problems with alcohol were reported (compared with only one person in both control groups). Table 19 details the types of trouble experienced. These teenagers had not yet been drinking heavily long enough to have experienced many of the social consequences of drinking, other than disordered family relationships. For example, only four pa-

TABLE 19

Problems with Alcohol among 110 Adolescent Psychiatric Inpatients

Type Problem	N
Never drank	44
Drank, never had problems	46
Drank, had problems*	20
Family objected to drinking	11
Patient thought he drank too much	11
Others thought he drank too much	8
Felt guilty about drinking	2
Lost friends because of drinking	0
Trouble at work or school because of drinking	3
Loss of job from drinking	1
Auto trouble from drinking	2
Arrested because drunk	2
Fighting because drunk	4
Benders (48 hours) more than once	1
Wanted to stop and could not	0
Drinking before breakfast	2
Amnestic episodes ("blackouts")	4
Impotence	0
Delirium tremens	2
Fearful while drinking	1

* Total number of problems was greater than the number of patients having problems (20), because of multiple type problems in some patients.

tients had had trouble with fighting while intoxicated, only two had had trouble with automobiles, and only two had been arrested.

Among the 110 psychiatric inpatients there was a history of inappropriate drug use (either the unprescribed use of prescription drugs or the use of illegal drugs) by 14 adolescents, six of whom had used such drugs excessively. Multiple use of drugs was the rule, and LSD, amphetamines, and marijuana were those most often employed. One well control admitted to drug experimentation, but no psychiatrically ill control did so.

Backgrounds of Psychiatric Inpatients, Psychiatrically Sick Controls, and Psychiatrically Well Controls

The three comparison groups were similar with respect to age, sex distribution, race, socioeconomic level, and intelligence. Systematic review of their life histories revealed a similar amount of ill health among the three groups (when all types of illnesses were considered together), similar interests and activities, similar types of home composition and family size, and similarity in the amount and severity of separation and bereavement experiences.

The majority of features in their backgrounds which *differentiated* psychiatrically ill subjects (whether or not they were in the psychiatric hospital) from psychiatrically well controls were attributable to two factors: first, there was a significantly higher rate of psychopathology, past or current, among the parents of the psychiatrically ill adolescents. And second, there was a history of more "premorbid" deviant scholastic and social behavior among the psychiatrically ill patients. As will be shown later, this misbehavior was characteristic of patients who were later to develop antisocial personality or a similar disorder, not of patients with affective disorders or schizophrenia.

REFERENCES

1. Morrison, J. R., Hudgens, R. W., and Barchha, R. G. Life events and psychiatric illness. Br. J. Psychiatry *114:* 423–432, 1968.
2. Reiss, A. J., Jr. *Occupations and Social Status.* New York, The Free Press of Glencoe, Inc., 1961.
3. Cadoret, R. J., Winokur, G., and Clayton, P. J. Family history studies: VII. Manic depressive disease *versus* depressive disease. Br. J. Psychiatry *116:* 625–635, 1970.
4. Robins, L. N. *Deviant Children Grown Up: A Sociologic and Psychiatric Study of Sociopathic Personality.* Baltimore, The Williams and Wilkins Company, 1966.
5. Murphy, G. E., Robins, E., Kuhn, N. O., and Christensen, R. F. Stress, sickness and psychiatric disorder in a "normal" population: a study of 101 young women. J. Nerv. Ment. Dis. *134:* 228–236, 1962.

4

Affective disorders

GENERAL CONSIDERATIONS

The affective disorders, depression and mania, are popular subjects of current psychiatric research. This is understandable, since such illnesses are quite prevalent in the general population. For example, on the basis of Helgason's careful epidemiologic study in Iceland,[1] Winokur and coworkers[2] calculated a morbid risk for all types of mood disorders of 5.39% for men and 9.19% for women, a rate which was seven to nine times higher than that for schizophrenia in the same population. Furthermore, with an increase in the availability of psychiatric services and the consequent treatment of people with moderate as well as severe illnesses, affective disorders now form the predominant category of psychiatric illness in inpatients and outpatients at many diverse types of treatment centers, ranging from private American services like Renard Hospital, the site of this study, to a public mental hospital in a small Central American country, Honduras.[3] In addition, patients with other disorders, not primarily affective in nature (for example, alcoholism, anxiety neurosis, hysteria, and chronic medical illnesses), often do not present for psychiatric treatment at all except during the episodes of depression which occasionally supervene in the course of those more chronic syndromes.

Another reason for the popularity of mania and depression as subjects for research is that they are usually remitting disorders. This gives investigators an opportunity to study the same patients in both the sick and well states. A third feature of affective illnesses which makes their study rewarding is that there are several factors or agents which favorably influence their course, for example, the passage of time, antidepressant drugs, electroconvulsive treatment, and lithium. Inquiry into the means by which these things effect changes in depression and mania have led to testable hypotheses about the nature and causes of the disorders, for instance, hypotheses concerning biologic rhythms, neurotransmitter substances in the brain, and so forth. More and more investigators naturally choose to follow up such promising leads.

If it makes sense to study affective disorders in general, it certainly makes sense to study them in teenagers. First of all, they occur in that age group in significant numbers: one-third of Winokur's group of 61 bipolar manic-depressives (patients with at least one episode of mania) had their first episode before age 20,[2] and 40% of Perris' bipolar probands had their first onsets between ages 15 and 25.[4] When unipolar patients (who have had only depression, never mania) are considered, or when bipolar and unipolar groups are considered together, a smaller proportion of the total have early onsets: only 10% of Perris' unipolar depressives were first ill between ages 15 and 25.[4] Although adolescents form only a minority of the patients admitted to Renard Hospital (9.7%) and an even smaller minority of those admitted with affective disorders, nevertheless, when an adolescent *is* admitted, the chances are about one in three that he suffers from primary depression or mania (Table 3 in Chapter 2). Even those who do not have primary affective disorder often show a prominent affective coloration to their symptom picture at the time of hospital admission. It is often the secondary intrusion of depressive symptoms into syndromes of other types which necessitates the admission of teenagers to a psychiatric hospital.

It is also useful to study affective disorders in teenagers as a basis for the longitudinal and family studies which can lead to more thorough understanding of the nature and classification of these illnesses. Such studies, investigating their subjects at more than one point in time, are freer of distortion and bias than cross-sectional studies, which depend on retrospective information for description of the course of an illness and of the temporal relationships between illness and social factors. If one begins with young patients, one has the opportunity for longer follow-ups, for observation of the effects of life experiences (including treatment) on the course of the illness and vice-versa, and for observation of distinct, perhaps atypical, manifestations of affective disorders in different epochs of the patients' lives.

CLASSIFICATION

Clinical studies of affective disorders have been numerous since the time of Kraepelin,[5] who systematically sorted out mania and depression from other forms of madness and described these illnesses in detail. Over the years since then, the diagnosis and classification of mania have not stirred much controversy, since mania is confined to the more easily recognizable bipolar (manic-depressive) affective disorder. But depression most often occurs in people who have never had mania, and workers have proposed a variety of classification systems for that syndrome. For example, classification has been based on severity (neurotic *vs.* psychotic depression),[6] symptom clusters (agitated *vs.* retarded),[7] presumed cause (endogenous *vs.* reactive),[8] age of onset (involutional depression),[6] presence or absence of a history of mania (unipolar *vs.* bipolar),[4] and presence or absence of a preexisting non-affective psychiatric illness (primary *vs.* secondary).[9]

Recently, Robins and Guze[9] reported a comprehensive review of longitudinal and family studies of affective disorders and summarized the evidence in favor of classifying depression according to potentially verifiable historic data: if the patient has never been sick before, or sick only with a previous affective disorder, he is called a "primary" depressive, otherwise he is called "secondary." This classification avoids the question of etiology, which cannot be identified with certainty, and deals with the questions of clinical complexity (does the patient have more than one type illness?) and chronology (which psychiatric syndrome came first in time?). The primary-secondary distinction also avoids implications inherent in the neurotic-psychotic or the retarded-agitated labels, namely, that a severe depression may be a different illness from a mild one, or that depressions with different symptom pictures may be different disorders.

Once a depressive illness is identified as primary, there is a rationale for further classifying it as either unipolar (the patient has never had mania) or bipolar (at least one episode of mania). Winokur, Clayton, and Reich[2] have given evidence that this is a valid distinction from their own case material and from that of other workers, for example, Perris.[4] On the basis of family studies, age of onset, and course of the disorders, unipolar and bipolar affective illnesses appear to be genetically and clinically distinct syndromes.

The primary-secondary and the unipolar-bipolar classifications of affective disorder were found applicable to the adolescent subjects in the present study. Before presenting our results, however, it is appropriate to review some of the literature on affective disorders in adolescents.

REVIEW OF LITERATURE

Systematic and detailed clinical studies of adolescent affective disorders and of sociologic and family backgrounds of the patients are seldom found in the English language literature. There have been numerous writings about adolescence as a time of life, with discussion of psychologic disturbances, including depressive *symptoms*. But the "syndrome" approach to disorders in teenagers has rarely been employed. Therefore, much of the available information on the specific subject of affective disorders must be gleaned from publications which deal with wider topics.

Many 19th century writers saw adolescence as a period of inevitable psychologic upheaval associated with sexual awakening and the increased demands of worldly responsibilities. Much of this work is not in English nor generally available in American libraries, but was reviewed in 1904 by Hall in two lengthy volumes.[10] This work is a presentation of Hall's own ideas about adolescence as a unique time of life and is a comprehensive survey of 19th century thinking about growth, development, child-rearing, education, and the physical and mental disorders of youth. The books contain much that now seems quaint or silly interspersed, however, with careful reviews of systematic clinical studies. One such study was published by Wille in 1898.[11] He stated that there was no special form of "adolescent psychosis" as had been stated by earlier investigators, but rather that all forms of known mental disorders might manifest themselves in this era of life, yet appear atypical in proportion to the youthfulness of the patients. Some investigations since have borne this out, and many psychiatrists today would probably find Wille's conclusions confirmed by their own clinical experience.

Certain more recent works regarding affective disorders in children and adolescents merit citation in some detail. Kasinin and Kaufman[12] in 1929 reported that only four of their 65 "psychotic" patients age 10 to 15 were manic-depressive. Later, Kasinin[13] reported 10 patients in this age group with affective psychoses, two with primarily a kinetic disturbance, hyperactive since infancy, and eight who had prominent mood disturbances, elation or depression. The outcome in the group was generally poor, with two becoming chronic invalids and eight making an "inferior" adjustment. In 1952, Despert[14] reported that only 26 of 400 children, age two to 16 years, in an outpatient clinic had predominantly depressive moods or suicidal preoccupations. He did not find suicide attempts linked with depression in this very young group, rather reporting that this was more often impulsive behavior. The issue of *The Nervous Child* in which Despert's article appeared was devoted to writings about affective disorders in childhood. In that same issue, Harms[15] reported ten cases of manic-depressive illness in children and attempted to explain the affective changes in terms of ego development and life experiences. He sought to prevent the full development of the illness by psychotherapy. By contrast, Campbell[16] has emphasized the hereditary and constitutional predisposition to bipolar affective disorder. In 1952, he reported six cases of mania and 12 of depression in children, with a family history of manic-depressive illness in 78%. He cited Kraepelin to the effect that one-sixth of first attacks in manic-depressives occur between ages 15 and 20.[16] In *Manic-Depressive Disease,* Campbell[17] said there was a premorbid cyclothymic personality in manic-depressive youngsters. He described in detail eight of 40 cases he had followed up. He stated that this disorder was often incorrectly diagnosed or erroneously attributed to environmental stresses. He believed that the illness was reversible with electroconvulsive treatment and deplored the tendency of so many psychiatrists to withhold ECT when it was indicated for the treatment of a youthful affective disorder.

In 1956, Sands[18] reported on 146 "psychotic" and "borderline psychotic" patients. The incidence of depression was one-third that of schizophrenia, although the author did not give precise figures. One-third of patients with depression had made suicide attempts. He stated that depressive mood was less fixed among these adolescents than among depressed adults and that in boys the symptoms were often covered by anxiety, in girls by "hysterical" symptoms. Eighteen of the unipolar depressed adolescents were followed up. After two to four years, 13 were well, 3 had had relapses, and 2 were "psychopathic." The exact figures regarding Sands' bipolar patients were not given, but he indicated that they had a good prognosis also.

Landolt[19] in 1957 reported a five- to 25-year follow-up of 44 of 60 circular manic-depressives (13 depressed, 47 overactive) who had been age 15 to 22 as index cases. Only 10 were well at follow-up, whereas 27 had continued cyclic episodes. Nine were diagnosed schizophrenic at follow-up (including two of the ten who recovered). All of these were called "catatonic," raising the possibility that some of them might have had depressive stupor instead of schizophrenia.

Olsen[20] reported a one- to 52-year follow-up (average 25 years) of 28 manic-depressive patients whose first attack had occurred before age 19. In these bipolar cases, 29% of whom had a manic-depressive parent, mania was four times as common as depression until age 18, but depression became equally frequent by age 23. The first attack in adolescence was "characterized by behavioral disturbances with pronounced antagonism to relatives." Sometimes the picture was initially thought to be encephalitis or a schizophreniform disorder. Some of Olsen's patients, although it is not clear how many, had frequent attacks during the early years after onset, but later "burned out" and had normal social adaptation. Social development was normal in 19 of the 28 patients, with subsequent recurrence and disability in late middle age in 10 of the 19. One patient committed suicide. About half the patients had premorbid (childhood) personalities characterized by "queerness" and "obstinancy." They did worse than the patients without abnormal personalities.

The above observations lead to the controversial question of whether there are identifiable precursors in childhood of bipolar affective disorder, and how often, if ever, the illness begins before puberty. A lucid discussion of this issue and the pertinent literature was presented by Anthony and Scott in 1960.[21] They offered strict criteria for diagnosing the disorder before puberty, including typical symptoms, course, and family history. They pointed out that a number of previous workers had indiscriminately labeled as manic-depressive some children who were merely hyperactive or affectively labile. Anthony and Scott then presented their own case, a boy with affective heredity on both sides of his family, who was first manic at age 12 and who pursued a circular course during the 10 years of follow-up. That patient, moreover, was reported to have had abnormally fluctuating moods since early childhood. In their discussion the authors departed from direct reporting and accounted for the onset of the disorder in their patient on psychodynamic grounds, with rather slender evidence to support that conclusion.

Carter,[22] in 1942, reported 78 "psychotic" patients aged 14 to 18, of whom 17 (22%) had affective disorder. After three years, 12 of the 17 were well, two were ill to a degree, but not hospitalized, and three had relapsed, requiring periodic rehospitalization. Five of the 17 cases had "schizophrenic traits," and only two of these recovered completely. Carter examined his material to discover prognostic factors in his entire group of 78 cases, rather than analyzing the case material by individual syndromes. He found that good prognosis was associated with acute onset, consonance of emotions with thought content, a stormy course of illness, disorientation, absence of persistent hallucinations, absence of somatic delusions, absence of "multiple hereditary tainting," stable parents, pyknic body type, good premorbid personality, and onset later in adolescence. It should be noted that most of these favorable prognostic factors are characteristic of affective disorder, as opposed to process schizophrenia.

Toolan[23] wrote that depression is fairly common among children and adolescents and may be underdiagnosed. In his case material, typical adult-type depression seldom occurred before age 16 or 17. However, he believed that depressive illness occurs even in infants, manifested by head-banging, and eating and sleeping disorders, and that in older children and early adolescents it may show up as apathy, temper tantrums, disobedience, and truancy. Long-term follow-up studies and systematic psychiatric studies of relatives will be needed before this hypothesis receives sufficient support.

Frommer,[24] who also believes depression to be a frequent childhood disorder, reported 32 cases of depression occurring in patients age nine to 15. One-third of their parents had had depression. Thirty of the patients had been depressed for more than a year, 8 for more than 5 years. This belied the clinical impression of some observers that early depressions are usually brief. Fifteen of Frommer's patients had prominent phobic symptoms, whereas in 16 the mood disorder itself was most notable. Sleep difficulty, abdominal pain, and headaches were prominent symptoms.

Poznanski and Zrull[25] reviewed 1788 child outpatient records, analyzing the data on 98 who were believed by the examiners to be at least moderately depressed. From these they selected 14 who fit their criteria for depression, but admitted that others of the 98 might have had the syndrome also. Six of 14 mothers of the patients had current depression and one father had committed suicide. Despite this, and despite the convincing picture of depression during interviews, these children had usually been referred for aggressive behavior. Twelve of the 14 demonstrated fighting and other destructive acts. (Their manifest psychopathology resembled more nearly that of children with early antisocial personality.) This is reminiscent of Toolan's "depressive equivalent," and like his data, can only be confirmed by follow-up.

King and Pittman[26] reported a six-year follow-up of 65 patients who had been 12 to 19 years old at the time of index admission. This was a series of consecutive admissions to Renard Hospital, the site of the current study. Twenty-six (40%) of the patients had affective disorder: six were bipolar and 20 unipolar. During the follow-up interval 13 (50%) of the patients were either symptom-free or had only brief, mild depressions. Seven had a severe single episode, and six had prolonged or multiple episodes. Despite recurrent illness in half the group, only three of the 26 had symptoms at the time of follow-up. The authors were impressed with the good prognosis of affective disorders, even among a sample hospitalized at such a young age. Most important, they demonstrated that classification of psychiatric patients by syndrome (*e.g.*, "depression," "antisocial personality," "schizophrenia," etc.) was better than a typologic classification ("neurotic," "psychotic," "behavior disorder"), in predicting course and outcome. Typologic categorization depended on severity or on the presence of acting-out, which might be a youthful feature of more than one syndrome. When a patient was sick during the follow-up interval, he could be classified according to the same syndrome, but manifest neurotic, psychotic, or primarily "behavioral" features at different times during his illness.

Annesley[27] reported a study of 362 hospitalized adolescents, only 15 of whom (4%) had affective disorder. Thirteen of these came from stable homes, and 13 were male. Five of the 15 were bipolar, 10 unipolar. Prognosis was good, with 12 recovered, two improved, and one unchanged two to five years after hospitalization. The low number of affective patients in Annesley's sample, and the high number of boys in the affective group raise the question as to whether this disorder was underdiagnosed.

Weiner has performed a service for students of the psychopathology of teenagers in *Psychological Disturbance in Adolescence*.[28] This book combines good clinical descriptions with a broad review of the literature. Like Toolan, Weiner found that depression is characterized by atypical patterns (for example, boredom, restlessness, acting-out) in early adolescence, and by recognizable adult patterns in the later teens. The author presented a clear discussion of differential diagnosis between depression and the three other major syndromes with which it is often confused in adolescents: organic brain dysfunction, antisocial personality, and schizophrenia.

A major recent study of teenagers is that of Masterson, summarized in *The Psychiatric Dilemma of Adolescence*.[29] He studied 101 psychiatric outpatients, age 12 to 18 (average age 16) and followed up 72 of them five years later. His 101 cases were selected from 227 applicants for admission to a clinic and represented the less sick and more cooperative portion of the total patient sample. Only 15% of the original 101 were ill enough to be called "psychotic," and only 11 of 78 patients received inpatient treatment during the follow-up period. He compared his probands with 101 controls who had never had psychiatric consultation, selected by random methods from the schools attended by the patients.

Two possible flaws in Masterson's study, the questionable representativeness of his samples and a somewhat bewildering mixture of syndrome classification with typologic classification, should not obscure the real importance of his book. For the author made a systematic attempt to classify every patient in some way and an attempt to assess the pathoplastic importance of the process of adolescence itself. The results of the first attempt are not wholly convincing, because some of his labels (*e.g.*, "passive-aggressive personality," "inadequate personality") do not represent well established symptom pictures. He might better have called these patients "undiagnosed" and adhered to classification according to established syndromes. But his attempt to deal with the clinical significance of adolescence has resulted in one of the major contributions to understanding psychiatric disorders in this confusing age group: the demonstration that the process of adolescence is not the essential factor in the psychiatric disorders of teenagers. It is true that he found that "adolescence" played a role in the clinical picture of 53 of 72 patients, as assessed by onset or worsening of illness during early adolescence and by "a clinical picture containing the elements of conflict known to be associated with this stage of the growth process," that is, new or intensified sexual or aggressive elements in the clinical picture. But it was the illnesses of the patients, neurosis, schizophrenia, or personality disorder, which dominated the picture, not the adolescent features, and the precursors of the disturbances often antedated the teenage years. The controls weathered adolescence without significant impairment unless a definite psychiatric disorder was present. And the sick subjects did not grow out of their illnesses after their adolescence terminated. "The decisive influence was psychiatric illness, not adolescent turmoil." Masterson was probably the first worker to demonstrate convincingly the misleading and imprecise nature of the term, "adolescent adjustment reaction."

Masterson's book is less helpful in dealing with affective disorders as such. Some depressives are classified in his "neurotic" group, and his case reports indicate that some patients who would be classified depressive in our study are in Masterson's schizophrenic group. (Evidently his criteria for schizophrenia are much broader that those used by us.) The manics, if any, are not in evidence. So it is difficult to trace the course and outcome of affective disorders in his case material. He does, however, identify a "depressive symptom pattern," which appears at follow-up in four of his 11 psychoneurotics and nine of his 18 schizophrenics, that is, in 18% of his total follow-up sample of 72 patients. This would seem a reasonable approximation of the incidence of depressive illness in this group of psychiatric outpatients. Twenty-four of his 43 patients with "personality disorder," presumably chronically disturbed, also had the depressive symptom pattern at follow-up. Possibly some of them corresponded to those psychiatric inpatients in our study whom we classified "undiagnosed, most like depression." Many of the latter had chronic problems with depressive symptoms, but were too atypical to be classified as definite depressives.

Finally, Masterson is in the company of a number of workers in adolescent psychiatry in his observation that psychopathology becomes more typical as the subjects grow older: "these patients, rather than showing unstable clinical pictures over the years, gradually tended to fit into more clearly differentiated and usual diagnostic categories." [29]

What, then, has been definitely established in the literature with regard to the specific subject of affective illness in children and adolescents? First, these disorders occur even in the prepubertal age group, although they are rare before age 14 or 15. There is controversy as to how prevalent they are, with some writers calling then unusual before adulthood and others reporting them as frequent. Second, the psychiatrically ill relatives of manic-depressive (bipolar) youngsters usually have manic-depressive illness themselves. Third, to the extent that a psychiatrically ill teenager's clinical picture is dominated by a disturbance of affect, rather than thinking or behavior, the illness tends to have a good prognosis for remission, although it may recur later. However, compared to *well* teenagers, those who have affective disorders during their adolescence may experience considerable impairment, not only from the illnesses themselves, but also from their occurrence at a critical time of life when so much is going on with respect to school, career choice, formation of peer-group relationships, and so forth. Fourth, the great majority of "average" teenagers weather the vicissitudes of these years without impairment by affective symptoms, although they encounter emotional stress during this epoch of life. Adolescence is not psychopathologic *per se,* and "adolescent adjustment reaction" is not a helpful label.

More controversy surrounds certain other findings in the literature. First, some writers state that affective disorders may be atypically expressed in teenagers, manifesting perhaps as a learning disorder, as transient antisocial behavior, or in other ways. Second, nothing definite has been established about premorbid personalities in young affective patients, although some workers suggest that a cyclothymic personality might be a frequent precursor of bipolar affective disorder. Third, there is evidence that schizophrenia has been overdiagnosed and affective disorders underdiagnosed by American psychiatrists in general.[30] The present author believes that this is especially the case where teenage patients are concerned. There has been a tendency to label as schizophrenic all severely ill adolescents, not only bizarre manics, but also the profoundly depressed adolescents who may be physically immobilized by their illness and burdened by delusions of guilt and worthlessness.

Finally, one thing that has not been established by studies to date is the specific cause, or causes, of manic and depressive illness. Affective heredity is one determinant of these disorders in many patients, but just how hereditary factors operate, or to what degree, is still unknown. The question of psychologic causation is even more cloudy, and deserves separate discussion.

LIFE EVENTS AND AFFECTIVE DISORDERS

There is no disputing the fact that many people who experience or anticipate personal catastrophe—for example, bereavement, imprisonment, or life-threatening illness—also experience severe emotional distress. They may call this distress "anxiety," "depression," "terror," "despair," or other words denoting dysphoric affect. There is also no disagreement that other people, experiencing the same catastrophic events, weather their storms with surprisingly little inner turmoil. Confronting this paradox, many investigators have postulated special factors of susceptibility in those who experience emotional breakdown under stress, and special protective factors in those who experience much less than the expected amount of distress under the blows of fate. But after at least 30 years of research in this area, there are still more questions than answers. In any case, it is well to remember that most people do not become severely disabled psychiatrically when terrible things happen to them, and that those who do become disabled regain their equilibrium in a reasonably short time. There is very little contention among psychiatric and sociologic researchers about these matters.

On the other hand, controversy has arisen concerning the reverse side of this issue—the role of stressful events in the genesis of sustained psychiatric disorders, especially affective illnesses. For many years there was widespread and uncritical acceptance of the thesis that nearly all disorders affecting the emotions could be traced to some meaningful personal experience or cluster of events, however farfetched or temporally remote the connection between the experience and the illness might appear by standards of common sense. There was a persistent assumption by many doctors that the *illnesses,* depression and mania, might simply be extensions of the *moods,* sadness and happiness. This seems logical when one is considering mild degrees of depression or hypomania, but less so in severe cases, when the clinical picture may include irrational judgment, delusions, hallucinations, bewilderment, and the extreme physiologic accompaniments of serious affective illness—immobility or frantic hyperactivity, intractable insomnia, profound loss of appetite, and so forth. Nevertheless, many clinicians (and patients themselves) have sought for causes of even such severe illnesses in the life events before onset, and until recently reports of such cause-effect relationships remained relatively unchallenged in the literature. Most, if not all, psychiatrists have experienced "certainty" in some of their cases that a given event triggered an episode of persistent affective illness. But anecdotal data and plausibility are not proofs of the truth of an assumption. In the past, some presumed causes of affective disorders have been shown to be consequences or symptoms of the illness (*e.g.*, lack of sleep "causing" depression or mania), and many positive studies have not only lacked controls, but have failed to take into account the fact that stressful events occur in everyone's life, and that by chance alone the onset of an illness will follow soon after some such event in a proportion of the cases.

In the past decade, however, the entire issue of the connection between life events and psychiatric illness has been reopened for critical investigation. Recent studies by Clayton,[31-33] Hudgens,[34-36] Brown,[37-41] Paykel[42, 43] and their co-workers, and by Holmes and Rahe[44, 45] have demonstrated a causal connection between stressful life events and subsequent worsening of conditions already underway, between life events and subsequent admission to psychiatric hospitals or clinics, and, in a substantial minority of bereaved persons, between bereavement and depressions of moderate degree for which psychiatric care was rarely sought. These investigations have not yet convincingly demonstrated (to the current author, at least) that life stress can cause madness in a person previously of sound mind, nor cause a severe depression sustained for many months and attended by multiple disturbances of physical and mental function.

A consideration of some methodologic necessities for a valid study of the relationship between stress and illness will demonstrate why there are so many difficulties in the interpretation of results, especially from retrospective studies. First, a valid study must date the onset of illness within a reasonable time span. This is extremely difficult to do, especially retrospectively, not only because the essence of a psychiatric illness cannot be specified, but also because early symptoms may be subtle or forgotten. Second, events must be dated, and anyone who has tried to do this retrospectively knows how difficult it is. Third, history must be replicated by informants. A study at our medical center comparing patients and their close relatives with respect to independent reporting of recent, specified stresses, showed significant discrepancies between informants' and patients' histories.[35] Fourth, there should be a quantification of the importance of each type of event for each patient: what is stressful for one person may be of little consequence to another. Fifth, diagnostically cohesive groups must be studied if any statement is to be made about precipitation of a specific syndrome. Sixth, a representative sample of people with a given syndrome must be considered if anything is to be said about the causes of such a disorder. Hospitalized patients are clearly not a representative sample of those with a given type illness; neither are outpatients, since care seeking is often determined by factors other than the occurrence of the illness; neither are cases found in house-to-house surveys, since in such surveys house-bound persons and women will be overrepresented and institutionalized persons will be missed. Seventh, the illness studied should be one that is demarcated by symptom type, severity, or duration from everyday emotional reactions that make sense in the context of the putatively causative events. Eighth, the same kind of event or cluster of circumstances which allegedly triggers an illness at one time in a patient's life should precipitate a recurrence later if the events recur in a similar context of emotional distress. Ninth, suitable control groups must be selected. There are possible problems with every type of control groups. For example, it can be objected that medically ill controls for a psychiatric study sample may themselves have illnesses precipitated by life stress. And it can be argued that general population controls for a psychiatric sample are *too* well, that the fact of illness and care seeking have not been held constant between the experimental and control groups, or that well controls are likely to underreport life stress because they worry less than psychiatric patients and have not had their memory refreshed by the repeated interviewing that is the fate of many psychiatric patients. Tenth, events that are possible consequences of the illnesses in question should be excluded from consideration as possible precipitants of the illness. Thus, the problems involved in studying, retrospectively, the relationship between multiple types of life events and the onset of psychiatric disorders are so great that the findings of such studies, whether positive or negative, will continue to provoke skepticism.

By contrast, the prospective study of the effect of a specific event, generally believed stressful, on a high risk population might have value. For example, Winokur, Clayton, and Reich[2] have reported that among their female manic-depressive patients, if a woman had ever had a postpartum episode, she invariably had a subsequent affective episode when she had another baby. The numbers were very small—three patients, six subsequent childbirths, and six recurrences of postpartum episodes—but the data suggest that it would be worthwhile to study this relationship prospectively in a large group of manic-depressive women of childbearing age. A testable hypothesis could be formed. If it were disproven it would not need repeated testing. If not disproven, this could lead to further studies, for example, on the nature of the event, parturition: emotional, endocrinologic, or so forth. These might someday lead to a discovery of "bridges" between the causative event and the essential internal changes that constitute affective disorder, whatever they may turn out to be.

In this way, knowledge about causation of affective disorders could be advanced, although investigation will continue for some time to be frustrated by certain basic problems inherent in studying psychiatric disorders. For example, as mentioned earlier, such disorders are usually describable only by history and by observation of behavior. Their "essence" is not known, and there are few biologic correlates of such disorders. And the organ generally considered most important in psychiatric symptom production is the brain, a most difficult object to study directly.

In any case, so far there has been no convincing scientific demonstration of a connection between life stresses and persistent affective disorders, but neither has such a connection been disproven. Most investigators, including the author, have the clinical impression that there *is* at times of cause-effect relationship between life stress and the onset of affective disorders in certain subjects with as yet poorly understood susceptibilities, genetic or experiential, and that people who are already psychiatrically ill may become worse at times of stress. Some supporting evidence for these impressions has been found in the current study among those adolescents hospitalized on non-psychiatric services who had depressions of moderate severity. This will be discussed later in this chapter.

AFFECTIVE DISORDERS IN THE CURRENT ADOLESCENT STUDY

Diagnostic Criteria

The following criteria were used to diagnose mania and depression in our sample:

Depression:

A. An onset, whether rapid or gradual, after which there was a difference from usual self, manifested predominantly by a dysphoric mood.

B. The change includes at least two of the following symptoms: self-blaming or self-negating attitude, diminished interest, excessive worrying, death wishes.

C. The change includes at least four of the following symptoms: anorexia, insomnia, decreased libido, tired, trouble thinking or concentrating, diminished or impaired activity, not keeping self well groomed, crying or other agitated behavior.

D. No disturbance of consciousness.

E. No other diagnosis likely to explain symptoms.

Mania:

A. An onset, whether rapid or gradual, after which there is a difference from usual self, predominantly manifested by a euphoric or frantic mood.

B. The change includes at least two of the following symptoms: inappropriately elated reaction to events, grandiose ideas about self, extreme impatience with restraint, excessive plans, excessive desire to spend money.

C. The change includes at least two of the following symptoms: overtalkativeness, thinking faster or changing subject rapidly, increased energy or physical activity, less sleep.

D. No disturbance of consciousness.

E. No other diagnosis likely to explain symptoms.

These criteria were developed in the Washington University Department of Psychiatry and took into account, especially, the prior work of Cassidy *et al.*,[46] and previous studies in this Department by Winokur[2] and Hudgens[3, 34] and their co-workers. The requirement that a patient be qualitatively different from his usual self in order to receive the research diagnosis of mania or depression was the key criterion. That is, there had to be a history of onset (although onset might have been quite gradual and long prior to admission) before which time the patient was free of the illness. The determination as to whether or not the patient was different from his usual self was made through direct questioning of the patients and their parents on this point and through the investigator's assessment of the entire history.

Those subjects whose clinical pictures resembled depression more than any other syndrome, but who failed to meet all the criteria for the diagnosis (either because of atypicality or sparsity of symptoms) are also considered in this chapter and called "undiagnosed, most like depression."

Totals with Affective Disorder or Possible Affective Disorder

Depression

In the current study there were 68 adolescents with definite or possible affective disorder.

Twenty-seven subjects, 19 psychiatric patients and 8 sick controls, received a diagnosis of definite depression by the research criteria. In 25 of the 27 definite depressives, the syndrome was "primary," that is, no other psychiatric illness preceded it in time; in the other two subjects the depressions were "secondary" in that they were preceded by sexual deviations (homosexuality in one case, foot fetishism in the other), which were in themselves troubling to the patients.

Among the 27 subjects with definite depression, two had previously had mania and 25 had not. Thus 25 of the depressives were unipolar, two were bipolar.

"Undiagnosed, Most Like Depression"

Twenty-eight adolescents, 14 psychiatric inpatients and 14 ill controls, were "undiagnosed, most like depression," that is, they had possible depression. Among these subjects, 25 had possible depression as their primary disorder, whereas three had epilepsy preceding the affective symptoms.

Mania

Eleven subjects, all of whom were psychiatric inpatients, were manic at the time of our study. None of them had had a prior psychiatric illness other than affective disorder, thus they were all cases of primary affective disorder. The 11 adolescents with mania, added to the two who were depressed at the time of our study but who had had mania in the past, made a total of 13 with bipolar (manic-depressive) affective disorder.

Optionally Classifiable Patients

One psychiatric inpatient was optionally classifiable as either depressed or alcoholic, and another psychiatric inpatient was optionally classifiable as either depressed or obsessive-compulsive (see Table 2, Chapter 2). Because of their complexity these last two cases will not be considered with the others in this chapter.

Bipolar (Manic-Depressive) Illness

Demographic and Family Data

Eight of the 13 manic-depressives were girls, five were boys. Twelve had never married, one was separated. Eleven were white, two black. At the time of the study, four patients were age 14 or 15, the other nine were 17 to 19. The average age was 17.2 years.

Seven of the 26 natural parents of the manic-depressives had a history of psychiatric disorders. Two fathers had unipolar depression, one was alcoholic, and one was undiagnosed. One mother had possible schizophrenia, one a unipolar depression, and only one had definite bipolar affective disorder. The apparently low incidence of manic-depressive illness among the psychiatrically ill parents of these bipolar patients was surprising, but it may turn out to be greater at follow-up. The three with unipolar depression may develop mania in the future, and the undiagnosed father may turn out to have manic-depressive illness when he is interviewed directly.

Only one manic-depressive adolescent had two psychiatrically ill natural parents, whereas five had one ill parent each. Thus 46% of the bipolar adolescents had at least one sick parent.

Premorbid Personalities

As mentioned earlier, some workers have made statements about premorbid personalities of young manic-depressives on the basis of histories taken at the time of illness. Such reports are suspect to some extent because of retrospective distortion by patients and families, the variability and selectivity of memory, and the absence of convincing criteria for classifying personality types. With respect to our own patients, no typical premorbid picture emerged, although this was systematically inquired about. Patients were usually described as psychiatrically healthy before onset. Examples of moodiness, extraversion, and misbehavior were reported, but the subjects could not be distinguished from well children and adolescents in this regard, even retrospectively. Five were described as relatively quiet, six as happy and active, and two had had behavior problems which were not unexpected in view of concurrent environmental circumstances.

Previous Episodes

The study admissions of the 13 manic-depressives were for treatment of a first episode in five cases. The other eight had had prior episodes. The first episode *ever* had been mania in seven patients, at an average age of 16.3 years (range 15 to 19) and depression in six patients at an average age of 15.3 years (range 14 to 18).

According to our best estimate the 13 manic-depressives had had, including the illness at the time of our study, a total of at least 15 manic episodes, nine depressions, and three mixed episodes (with manic and depressive symptoms both very prominent in the same episode). If the mixed episodes are scored as manic, there were twice as many "manias" as "depressions" in our subjects, and an average of two episodes of any type for each patient. This compares with the data of other workers, including Olsen[20] who found mania four times as common as depression prior to age 18. We believe there may be a general tendency on the part of patients and relatives to underreport depressive episodes retrospectively, since they are less memorable than manic episodes and, if relatively mild, are less likely to result in hospitalization or complaints by schools and parents.

Looking back on the histories of those patients who had had prior episodes, it was possible to decide retrospectively whether or not a patient had been disabled at home or school by affective symptoms at a given time in the past. Since the presence of disability was one of our previously established criteria for scoring affective symptoms as an "episode," it was always possible to distinguish times of "illness" from times of "wellness" by our own definition. But one should not be entirely comfortable with this: severe manic and depressive episodes may be preceded by what looks for a time like appropriate elation or sadness. No one can be sure that transient, non-impairing moodiness in a teenager with a prior history of bipolar affective disorder is not a "micro-episode," qualitatively like the illness itself. There is no test for the presence of affective illness, except for severity of symptoms, inappropriateness of symptoms relative to life events, persistence of symptoms, or disability.

The Clinical Picture of Mania

General Considerations. The clinical picture of depression among bipolar patients did not differ from that of patients with unipolar affective disorder. For this reason, the symptomatology of mania will be described in the current section of the chapter, and depression will be considered only in the section on unipolar affective disorder.

The reader should keep in mind that all our study patients were hospitalized, thus were examples of the more ill manic-depressive teenagers. Many bipolar patients never enter the hospital if they are not more than hypomanic while in the "high" phase or not suicidal while depressed. Some of our patients had had such milder episodes previously.

Onset. The mode of onset in mania may be gradual or abrupt, and the clinical picture may range from moderate euphoria and silliness, to an agonized, deluded frenzy. The rapidity with which manic symptoms developed in our patients and mounted in intensity determined the interval between onset and hospitalization. The sooner a patient got into treatment, the better things went for him. So, in a sense, fortune favored a teenage manic who had the sudden onset of a flagrantly psychotic state that resulted in immediate hospitalization. By contrast, a patient who had a prolonged hypomanic phase, not so dramatic nor so readily identifiable as illness, might not be brought to treatment early enough, and might get into considerable difficulty because of the consequences of hyperactivity and poor judgment. Two cases will illustrate this contrast:

> *032*—A patient with rapid onset was a 15-year-old white girl with a stable premorbid personality who had been well until two days before hospital admission. At that time, while with friends and on no drugs, she began to write a play which was to be used at a farewell party for the minister of her church. The writing was noted by her friends to be nonsensical, and was placed at odd angles on the pages. She herself said that she was doing research into the use of popular music for religious purposes. The next day at school she appeared

bewildered and wandered about, leaving her books in the wrong classroom. The faculty noticed that she was preoccupied, laughed inappropriately, and spoke irrationally. Her parents were called and took her to a local hospital, whence she was admitted to Renard Hospital the following day. She was elated, with push of speech, laughed and joked inappropriately, and was very distractable during the interview. For example, at the sound of footsteps outside her room she interrupted the interviewer with "That's Ed going by now! Whoosh! You wouldn't *believe* the things he does!" She recurrently referred to local radio shows and popular groups of musicians, out of the context of the interview.

The above patient became bizarrely ill quickly enough that she received immediate psychiatric inpatient treatment, and little harm resulted from the episode. By contrast, the patient below suffered considerable and prolonged social difficulty and embarrassment.

014—At the age of 15, four and a half years before the study admission, this white girl had the onset of a depression with lethargy, inability to complete school and home tasks, feelings of worthlessness, and thoughts of suicide. These subsided spontaneously in four months. She remained well until 26 months later, age 17, when she developed argumentativeness, excessive drinking, and sexual promiscuity. Her drinking resulted in expulsion from high school, and her promiscuity, elation, and emotional lability continued for about six months. This phase was succeeded by four months of depression and apathy, with no sexual activity, which was in turn followed by a recurrence of mania: increased activity, elation, loudness, irritability, and open, indiscriminant solicitation of sex from boys. This phase lasted three months before her family sought psychiatric help. Her illness, identified by her associates as "bad behavior," resulted in serious impairment of her social reputation and her educational advancement, loss of most of her friends, and alienation from her bewildered family. (Over the succeeding years, while maintained on lithium therapy, this patient slowly rebuilt her life, socially and professionally. Her younger sister subsequently developed circular manic-depressive illness at age 15; but she received immediate treatment, and such devastating consequences were averted.)

Among the 11 manics immediate hospitalization was not the rule. Only one was hospitalized within a week of onset of the episode of illness. Four were hospitalized within a month, eight within three months, and all 11 within six months after onset.

The Clinical Picture of Mania at Height of Illness: Diagnostic Difficulties. When a patient was very ill, it was often not possible to make the diagnosis of mania by taking the history from him alone and observing his mental status. In the first place, patients typically had little insight into the fact that their mood and behavior were abnormal, although most acknowledged that their own actions had led to their restriction to a hospital environment: "I am tired from working too hard, and I need a rest," or "Maybe I am in the hospital to heal people, I'm not sick." In the second place, retrospective distortions of the history were the rule. One patient, manic for only a few days, said that God had been controlling her for five years. It was not unusual for patients to feel that the current euphoric state represented their "real selves" being expressed for the first time in their lives. In the third place, the cross-sectional clinical picture at the time of admission, observed without benefit of reliable longitudinal history, could resemble depression, schizophrenia, or organic brain syndrome, and even sociopathy or hysteria. The symptomatology was often quite bewildering. So it proved of the utmost importance to take a systematic history from a reliable informant who had known the patient for some time. Mania could not be diagnosed unless *the changes represented differences from the patient's usual self,* and this could not reliably be determined merely by talking to the patient. Furthermore, the changes had to occur *in the predominant context of a euphoric or frantic mood.* For example, auditory hallucinations, when present, were typically ephemeral, and much less notable than the mood disturbance; and antisocial acting-out was temporally confined to circumscribed periods of hyperactivity. These facts could not be determined by talking only to the patient while he was sick.

Table 20, which lists symptoms which were present in more than a third of the adolescents during their manic episodes, demonstrates the complexity of the clinical picture. It is most important to realize that mania is not exclusively a mood disorder, although this factor is predominant. There may be disturbances of behavior, thought process, thought content, intellectual function, memory, orientation, vegetative functions (*e.g.,* sleep, appetite, sex drive), and perception (hallucinations, increased intensity of sensory experience, and so forth). Moreover, the mood disorder itself may vary from elation to extreme anger; and transient depressive affect with suicidal ideas occurred briefly in almost half the manic episodes in the present study. Suicide attempts, however, are not a feature of mania, and occurred in none of our patients' episodes. Concern about the possibility of suicide was not spontaneously mentioned, by either patients or parents, as a reason for the hospital admission of any manic.

TABLE 20

Symptoms Occurring in Manic Episodes

	N = 11
	%
Elation	91
Sense of strength, importance	73
Other grandiose ideas	73
Overtalkativeness	73
Nervousness	64
Trouble thinking	64
Depressed mood	64
Faster thoughts	64
Less need for sleep	55
Problems sleeping	55
Feelings of unreality	45
Auditory hallucinations	45
Thoughts of suicide	45
Increased libido	45
People watching	36
People plotting	36
Wanting to die	36
Decreased appetite	36
Crying	36

Nonetheless, patients who are manic may have a typical depressive episode following the subsidence of mania. Then, of course, suicide must be considered a possibility.

That a patient may be quite psychotic, yet still manic-depressive, as determined by the longitudinal picture and the typical mood disturbance, is demonstrable in that, at times, five of our 11 manics had auditory hallucinations, four had delusions of being plotted against, three had delusions of thought control, and three had visual hallucinations. In fact, such symptoms and the attendant fear or bewilderment could dominate the clinical picture transiently: hyperactivity and push of speech need not be present during every hour of the illness to sustain a diagnosis of mania.

Somatic complaints were rare, and only two of the eleven patients were classified as heavy drinkers at the time of the manic episode.

The following case illustrated the complexity that is possible in the clinical picture of acute mania:

013—Premorbidly, this white girl was described by her father as "normal, vivacious, and easy to work with." One month before her first psychiatric hospital admission at age 15, after a long hike at camp, she developed déjà vu feelings, and thoughts about the history and geography of the camp kept intruding in her mind. After that she was nervous, worried about schoolwork, and experienced fast thoughts. Her symptoms did not come to others' attention, however, until four weeks after onset, three days before admission. At that time she began to talk in a high-pitched voice, stare fixedly at the ceiling, and respond slowly to conversation. She then began to believe that a professional football player on television and her own dog were sending messages to her. She heard footsteps in the house when no one else did, became frightened, and told her father to carry a gun for protection. She told her parents that she was going to California to enter the Miss Teenage America contest, and that her father was to go to Washington to testify about the Ku Klux Klan. She would act as a decoy for her father to protect him. Her speech became more and more pressured and irrational. The next day, while driving with her parents, she mistakenly said that strangers on the street were people known to her, and she waved to them.

Upon admission to the hospital she exhibited push of speech and flight of ideas, but no motor hyperactivity. Almost all responses to questions appeared irrelevant. She was oriented to place and time and elated upon admission, but on the next day developed hyperactivity, disrespectfulness, distractibility, echopraxia, and echolalia. She could hear the voice of her family doctor calling her. She responded rapidly to lithium carbonate, however, and was discharged after 10 days, essentially asymptomatic.

For the three next months she was well, happy, and not impaired in schoolwork. Then, three days before her second admission (the study admission), she began to be overly amused and silly. She developed heightened interest in boys, but did not act out sexually. She became distractible, ideas suddenly appearing in her mind, and she heard voices faintly and transiently as if from a distance. On admission, she demonstrated silly affect, but no push of speech or hyperactivity. During her hospitalization, she once more received lithium carbonate. Periods of hyperactivity recurred before lithium took effect, and their subsequent occurrence coincided with low blood levels of lithium. She recovered and was discharged in 23 days.

Disorders in adolescents for which mania may be most often mistaken, and vice-versa, are encephalitis or other neurologic conditions, drug reactions, and schizophrenia. From a practical standpoint, once a teenager is sick enough to require hospital admission, encephalitis is not difficult to distinguish from mania. Even when encephalitis presents with a frenzied, manic-like picture, the physician is not likely to miss the diagnosis for more than a day or two if he thinks of the possibility and observes the patient for the presence of headache, fever, altered consciousness, persistent confusion, and spinal fluid abnormalities. Other organic brain disorders (for example, tumors), should be productive of neurologic signs or abnormal results from diagnostic procedures by the time they have progressed to the extent of producing a prominent mental disturbance.

Drug reactions may at times be confused with mania, especially in an outpatient whose mental status and behavior are not under daily observation by the physician, and who cannot be kept from receiving drugs "on the street." Once a patient is in the hospital these factors present much less of a problem, although patients who are determined to do so can succeed in having drugs smuggled in to them, even on a locked psychiatric ward. The effect of hallucinogens, for instance, LSD and mescaline, may transiently resemble mania in all respects, but typically subside in less than 24 hours. Amphetamines, the most frequently abused type of CNS stimulants, can produce agitation, euphoria, perceptual disorders, and delusions of a paranoid type. If the patient stops taking the drug, he typically experiences a physical and emotional letdown, and the psychotic symptoms usually subside within a few days. The urine can be tested for the presence of amphetamines also.

The greatest problem in differential diagnosis of mania is to distinguish the condition from schizophrenia. Among our 110 psychiatric inpatients there were 11 manics, 6 schizophrenics, one "undiagnosed, like schizophrenia," and 7 patients in whom we could not decide between affective disorder and schizophrenia. These adolescents were labeled "undiagnosed, schizoaffective." They did not qualify for the manic label (despite the acuteness of their illnesses and the presence of definite affective symptoms) because of the prominence of behavior and thought content which were not logically consonant with affective disorder, or because of a dominance of hallucinations in the clinical picture. Previous studies of larger groups of such patients suggest that many of them have manic-depressive illness as determined at follow-up by the fact that their illnesses remit, that they later have typical episodes of depression or mania, and that they have a high incidence of affective disorders among near relatives.[47, 48] Nonetheless, a minority of such patients do turn out to have schizophrenia at follow-up, and it is not possible to be certain, early in the course of such bizarre illness in such young persons, which patients will have which outcome.

Course of Mania. Mania typically progresses to recovery, and responds symptomatically to lithium, phenothiazines, and electroconvulsive treatment. Only one of the 11 manic adolescents in this study received ECT on the index admission. On medication, our subjects improved significantly, usually within two weeks, though they were seldom ready for discharge that soon.

In the controlled hospital environment, push of speech and hyperactive behavior as a rule subsided before the mood had returned to normal and before good judgment had been reestablished. This could deceive the physician into thinking that the adolescent was more well than he in fact was, especially if the doctor had not known the patient before he developed mania.

The length of index hospitalization for the 11 manics ranged from 8 to 131 days (median patient, 23 days; mean, 35 days). Four manics were hospitalized from eight to 11 days, five from 22 to 41 days, one for 69 days, and one for 131 days. But this does not tell the entire story about the length of the index episodes. Even though the current study does not include systematic follow-up after study hospitalization, information already available demonstrates that at least eight of the 13 bipolar patients were discharged from the hospital too soon, as determined by the fact that their symptoms had not fully subsided and that they were later readmitted for treatment of the same episode. In two cases the study admission was a readmission for the same episode. In seven cases, including one of the above, readmission was necessary after the study hospitalization. Thus no more than five of the 13 bipolar adolescents escaped a fate of double or triple hospitalization for the same episode. Even some of those five patients may have been readmitted elsewhere; we only know they were not readmitted to Renard Hospital.

Table 21 summarizes the information concerning readmission. Five of the seven manics "rebounded" into worsened mania upon discharge,

TABLE 21

Data Concerning Rehospitalization during Current Episode of Manic-Depressive Illness

(Eight of 13 patients were rehospitalized)

Patient	Phase of Illness during Initial Admission	Phase of Illness for Which Readmitted	Duration of Hospitalization Which Preceded Readmission	Interval between Discharge and Readmission
			days	*days*
Y-014	mania	mania	11	18
Y-021	mania	mania	10	37
Y-029*	mania	mania	21, 131	20, 19
Y-032	mania	mania	8	6
Y-056	mania	depression	32	32
Y-078	mania	mania	8	4
Y-087	depression	depression	21	14
Y-105	mania	depression	22	14

* Had three admissions for same episode, one preceding the study admission and one following it.

whereas two developed abrupt depressions. One depressive was readmitted for depression. For six of the eight patients, the readmission occurred within three weeks of discharge.

Excluding the one admission of 131 days, the eight adolescents admitted more than once during the study episode had a mean length of admission of 17 days (range eight to 32 days), whereas the five patients not readmitted (presumably adequately treated) were in the hospital an average of 36 days (range 15 to 69 days). Perhaps two weeks is simply too short a period of inpatient treatment for a manic-depressive adolescent who is sick enough to require admission.

It seems likely that the apparent "double-peaked" course of illness in our manic adolescent subjects was an artifact either of premature release from the discipline of the hospital environment or of failure to take medication (usually lithium) as an outpatient. It may also have been a consequence of the usual practice at Renard Hospital of not giving ECT to manic teenagers.

Unipolar (Depressive) Illness

Demographic and Family Data

There were 25 subjects (17 psychiatric inpatients and eight sick controls) who had a diagnosis of definite depression by our criteria and who had never had mania. Twenty-four of these adolescents had depression at the time of the study, one (a control) had had only a past episode. There were 11 boys and 14 girls. Four subjects were married, 21 single. One was black, 24 white. The average age was 17.6 years at the time of admission (range 14 to 19). Sixteen of the 25 patients were 18 or 19 years old.

Seventeen of the 50 natural parents (34%) had a history of psychiatric disorder. Two fathers and five mothers had depression; four fathers were alcoholic, two mothers hysterics, and two mothers and two fathers were undiagnosed. In all, 58% of the depressed adolescents had at least one natural parent with a history of psychiatric illness. Three subjects had two sick parents each, while 11 had one sick parent.

Premorbid Personalities

It was among the unipolar depressive patients rather than the bipolars (manic-depressives) that indications of premorbid psychiatric abnormalities were found. Twelve of the 25 had a history, obtained independently from patients and parents, of recurrent affective symptoms persistent for years before the clear onset of the syndrome of disabling depression. For example, they were described as moody at times, obsessional, easily discouraged or upset, and three had had recurrent thoughts of suicide for years. As mentioned earlier, such reports of the premorbid state must be viewed with reservation, since they were retrospective, but in the current study these reports were convincing to the interviewers. Thus, among almost half of the unipolar depressives, the illness arose in youths with apparent affective instability, although the depressive illnesses themselves were demarcated from the pre-existing personality by numbers of symptoms and the onset of definite disability. Follow-up of these patients into adulthood should be especially interesting, since they would seem less likely to have long symptom-free periods than the group without premorbid instability. Whether or not they become addicted to drugs and alcohol, or develop other chronic disorders (besides depression) remains to be seen.

Of the 12 patients with premorbid affective symptoms, the symptoms were associated with sexual deviation in two and chronic medical conditions in two others. One example of each follows:

> Y-005—This 17-year-old white boy began to rub his parents' feet at age six or seven, because he liked the smell. He experienced no sexual excitement from this at first. At age 11 or 12, however, he began to masturbate with sexual fantasies about boys' stockinged feet. He began to rub his classmates' feet in school and would get an erection when he did. His classmates thought him "queer," he stated, but they let him rub their feet. He felt chronically guilty and odd because of this, and since his preteen years he had been nervous and thought of suicide. At age 16, he developed an episode of irritability, sustained depression, and worry about sexual desires for another boy. He was treated as an outpatient with chlorpromazine and reassurance, and he improved in two months. Three months after recovery, however, the depression returned. He felt "numb, void, bumbling, out of place." He started to quarrel with his parents. Suicide began to seem a logical alternative to his distress. The night before admission, after a month or so of depression, the patient took 52 over-the-counter sleeping tablets and left a note for his parents: "Try to understand. Forgive me, I love you." He awoke several hours later with stomach cramps, called to his mother, and was taken to the hospital.

> Y-016—This 18-year-old white girl had had an operation for scoliosis at age 15 with insertion of a rod along the vertebral column. She was then in bed for 6 months and was at times nervous and discouraged about her medical condition. These moods recurred periodically but briefly. At age 17, although medically well, she developed inability to do schoolwork, obsessional worrying over trivia, and despondency.

These symptoms increased in severity over a period of 10 months, at which time she attempted suicide twice within a week (ingesting aspirin, then iodine), telling no one about it at the time. On Christmas Eve, 16 days later, her mind "a blank," she wandered into a stable near her home and lay down, feeling "it was no use. I just gave up." It was winter, and she was very cold, but did not want to move and took no food or water. She was found 60 hours later, after a widespread search by police and volunteers, and was admitted to the hospital.

Previous Episodes

Of the 17 psychiatric inpatients, 12 were in the hospital for treatment of their first episode of depression, whereas five had had one prior episode. Of the eight controls, one was well at the time of the study, and seven were having their first episode of depression during the study admission. The controls, however, were in the hospital for medical and surgical treatment, not because of depression, which was an incidental finding.

For the 25 depressives, the onset of the first episode ever of depression was at a mean age of 15.9 years, an average of 1.7 years prior to the study admission (range 10 to 19 years; median age 16). Three of the patients had had the first onset before age 12, two others at age 14. Thus there was a tendency for unipolar depression (as well as the depressive phase in our bipolar patients) to begin earlier than mania. An example of very early onset follows:

Y-077—This 16-year-old white boy, a native of Cuba residing in the U.S. since early childhood, was well until age 10, although prior to that he had felt self-conscious and anxious in school because of early language problems. At age 10 he developed depressed mood, fatigue, anxiety, crying spells, and fear of failure. He hoped the car would wreck, killing him. He began to ruminate obsessionally over trivia, for example, greasy chicken that had spilled on the floor, or an unclean toilet. He could not concentrate on his school work because of such thoughts. Sometimes when listening to the radio, he would think of sin. He recovered after a few months and several psychotherapy sessions. (This information was available from the records of a psychiatric clinic the patient attended at age 10.)

From age 10 until 16, he was well except for occasional very brief periods of sadness, tension, and obsessional thoughts. He was extremely effective in school and in his extracurricular activities.

At age 16 he was placed in a slower group in one of his subjects at the beginning of the school year. He became anxious, worried that he might be stupid, and restricted his social life and extracurricular activities in order to study. Over the next two months he became increasingly tense and worried. He began to have crying spells, lost confidence in himself, and repeatedly sought reassurance from his parents. He developed a compulsion to look at objects over and over again. About two weeks before this study admission, after he had been sick for two months, he began to sit for long periods of time, blinking his eyes, and saying over and over "It's no use. It's no use." He began to drive the car very fast at times with suicide in mind, but did not hit anything. Once he lay down inside his parked car with the motor running, hoping that carbon monoxide would kill him, but he changed his mind. He was admitted after two weeks of unsuccessful treatment on antidepressants.

Where depression was concerned it was difficult to ascertain precisely the times of onset or the duration of prior episodes, unless old psychiatric records were available. Among patients with brief, recurrent, non-disabling affective symptoms the illness itself could begin gradually over a period of weeks or months, presenting initially as an exaggeration of pre-existing personality traits. However, all 25 subjects in our study who were diagnosed as definite unipolar depression were distinctly different from their usual selves at the times of their illnesses and had multiple symptoms fulfilling our criteria for the disorder. As mentioned, 20 (12 psychiatric patients, all eight controls) had only one episode in their lives, whereas five psychiatric patients had two episodes, including the illness at the time of our study.

The Clinical Picture of Depression

Onset. As a rule the onsets of episodes of depression were gradual, building up over a period of weeks or months. Early symptoms of depression, unlike those of mania, were usually undramatic and were initially ascribed by patients and parents to commonplace moodiness or to environmental circumstances. It was only after symptoms persisted for weeks, were severe, or seemed illogical in terms of life events that psychiatric help was sought. Only the 17 psychiatric patients were currently under treatment for depression. The seven controls who were depressed at the time of the study were in the hospital for other conditions. These two groups should be considered separately with respect to events leading to hospitalization.

Among the 17 depressed psychiatric inpatients, there was typically a long interval between the onset of depression and inpatient treatment for that condition. Only three patients (18%) had been ill for less than three months before admission. Eight had been ill from three to six months, two from six to 12 months, and four longer than a year. Hospitalization was thus not so rapid as for the manic subjects, 73% of whom were hospitalized within three months of onset. It was the rule for depressives to come to treatment later than manics, since their onsets were more gradual and less bizarre, and to have a period of unsuccessful outpatient treatment before hospitalization.

Of course, various life stresses, particularly in the interpersonal sphere (*e.g.*, with parents), accompanied the illnesses. This is demonstrably true in the course of all psychiatric disorders. However, it is uncertain, as mentioned earlier, whether life events played an etiologic role in the precipitation of illness. In any case, none of our 17 depressed psychiatric inpatients had life stresses which were objectively so severe as to make subsequent sustained depressive illnesses seem a "natural" consequence. The situation was different with respect to the depressed controls, who had milder forms of illness. This will be discussed later in this chapter.

The decision to hospitalize a depressed teenager was frequently precipitated by a suicide attempt. Ten of the 17 psychiatric inpatients (76%) had made at least one attempt, and three had made two attempts. The most recent attempt was within a week of hospitalization for four of the attempters, within a month for six (60%). The issue of suicidal behavior will be explored in the next chapter. Such actions are currently major reasons for psychiatric hospitalization of adolescents in this country, whatever the diagnosis.

The Clinical Picture of Depression at the Height of the Illness: Diagnostic Difficulties. Table 22 lists the common symptoms of depression in three studies: the current one, and two studies of adult inpatients by Cassidy *et al.*,[46] and Woodruff *et al.*[49] The latter investigation was conducted at Renard Hospital, the site of our research. The Cassidy and Woodruff studies both used criteria for depression similar to ours. In Table 22, the adolescent controls are listed separately from the adolescent psychiatric inpatients, since the former were not under treatment for depression. Hence, they were not a comparable group with respect to severity or numbers of symptoms.

Symptoms are listed in five categories: affective changes, suicidal symptoms, thinking disorder, changes in function or behavior, and physical symptoms. Any symptom which occurred in at least 48% of any patient group was listed. It should be noted that not every patient was scored as "depressed" or "sad." The patients did not need to describe themselves exactly in that way in order to be scored as having dysphoric affect. Other symptoms, notably nervousness and pessimism, could serve to fulfill that criterion for the diagnosis.

Inspection of the table reveals that the depressed controls, hospitalized on medical, surgical, and pediatric wards, were not as ill as the psychiatric

TABLE 22

Common Symptoms of Depression in Adults and Adolescents
(Dashes indicate the questions were not asked)

Symptom	Adolescent Psych. Inpts. N = 19*	Adolescent Controls N = 8	Adult Psych. Inpts., age 23–79 mean 48 years (Cassidy, *et al.*[46]) N = 100	Adult Psych. Inpts., age 21–65 mean 42 years (Woodruff, *et al.*[49]) N = 54
	%	%	%	%
I. Affective changes				
Depressed, sad	95	63	95	93
Loss of interest	79	63	—	89
Hopelessness	89	25	—	61
Nervous	74	38	—	—
Worry	63	63	—	—
Worthless	63	38	—	74
Guilty	63	25	—	28
Self a burden to others	58	25	—	—
Pessimism, not get well	53	12	—	61
Fear losing mind	—	—	63	—
Self reproach	—	—	—	59
II. Suicidal symptoms				
Want to die	89	50	—	—
Thought of suicide	84	50	45	41
Talked of suicide	58	38	—	—
Suicide attempt	68	0	—	11
III. Thinking disorder				
Trouble concentrating	84	63	83	93
Memory disturbed	53	25	52	—
Thinking slowed	—	—	64	69
Indecisive	—	—	—	59
IV. Function, behavior				
Task disability	89	38	—	78
Any insomnia	74	50	94	—
Trouble going to sleep	63	50	72	59
Restless sleep	63	12	56	46
Early a.m. awakening	32	0	80	61
Decreased sex	—	—	63	50
"Spells" †	—	—	62	—
Crying	32	63	72	50
Irritable	42	12	75	67
Restless	—	—	—	59
V. Physical symptoms				
Anorexia	74	38	88	87
Tired, weak	58	50	54	57
Palpitations	53	25	57	—
Weight loss	53	12	73	87
Nausea	21	25	48	—
Dyspnea	16	38	77	—
Constipation	16	12	60	28
Urinary frequency	—	—	60	—
Headaches	42	50	49	—
Paresthesias	—	—	53	—
Muscular tension	—	—	—	61

* "Adolescent psychiatric inpatients" includes the two bipolar patients who were depressed on index admission.

† "Spells" include anxiety attacks, dizzy spells, confused spells, and syncope.

inpatients. This was due to a selection factor, as mentioned. But the most notable finding in Table 22 is the similarity between the adults and adolescent psychiatric inpatients with respect to the clinical picture of depression. Our diagnostic criteria, then, served to select a typical depressive group, who resembled adult depressed patients not only with respect to affective symptoms, but with respect to physical and functional symptoms as well. The most notable differences between the younger and older samples were the significantly greater amount of suicidal thoughts ($p < 0.001$) and attempts ($p < 0.001$) among the teenagers. This finding will be discussed in Chapter 5.

Examination of this group of teenage depressives does not resolve the question of whether this disorder often presents atypically during adolescence. Our sample of definite depressives was selected for typicality. If this question is to be answered by this study, it will be answered only after studying "undiagnosed" patients at follow-up. In this study there is slender evidence to support the concept of "depressive equivalents" in youngsters. Investigators might be well advised to confine the use of the diagnosis, depression, to fairly typical cases. They do occur among teenagers.

Compared to mania, the diagnosis of depression is not so difficult to make at first contact, if one has a complete history. Of course, it is essential to talk to a knowledgeable informant, especially in very sick cases, as the patients are often so influenced by their current mood and thinking that they distort the past history in the light of their present pessimism and distress. It may seem to the patient that he has "always" been worthless, sad, incompetent, and so forth. But discussion with a parent may reveal that the disability is of recent origin. The patient may temporarily attribute greater significance to bad things in his past, while forgetting or undervaluing the good things. When patients recover, their sense of proportion about the past is usually restored. Similarly, the depressed patient is usually more keenly aware of interpersonal conflicts and may exaggerate them. While he was depressed, one 16-year-old boy viewed his father as especially overbearing and his mother as querulous. These features were present to some extent in his parents as constant factors, but before his illness and after his recovery the boy coped successfully with their undesirable traits. While he was sick, he wanted to talk about these character traits a great deal, believing they might have caused his illness; after he recovered, they did not seem especially relevant to him.

In the teenager (or adult) who is sick enough with depression to be hospitalized, the illness affects broad areas of his life. It is dominated, of course, by dysphoric affect, a qualitative and quantitative change from his usual self; and suicidal thoughts and overt suicidal communication or behavior are the rule. But thinking is affected also, with disturbed concentration and memory, and physical complaints and functional disability are prominent. Distortions of thought content and judgment may reach delusional proportions, especially in the area of guilt feelings and ideas of worthlessness. A severely depressed adolescent may be as socially inaccessible, withdrawn, or stuporous as a 65-year-old patient with the same disorder, and he will then need the same treatment.

By contrast with mania and schizophrenia, hallucinations were rare. Only one of our 27 adolescent depressives had auditory hallucinations, and one had visual hallucinations. Only one of Woodruff's 54 depressed adults was hallucinated at the time of that study;[49] and seven of Cassidy's 100 inpatients had hallucinations during their illnesses.[46] Depressive "voices" were transitory, usually located in the head, and were typically single words or accusatory fragments of sentences.

None of the 27 adolescent depressives (25 unipolar, two bipolar) considered in this chapter had abused drugs or alcohol,* but this was in part a selection factor. The abuse of such substances can so dominate the clinical picture as to override the importance of affective symptoms. That may have been the case in some of our patients who were labeled "undiagnosed, unclassified" (Chapter 8). Affective symptoms were very prevalent among patients in the latter category, as will be shown, and some may have had underlying depressions.

In general, drug abuse is a disorder which may be confused with depression. Only a careful history from several sources (including peers) and observation of the patient in the drug-free state can establish the diagnosis of depression and rule out drug abuse. Schizophrenia, which is unfortunately overdiagnosed by many American psychiatrists in many very sick teenagers with whatever illness, should seldom be confused with depression, if the diagnostic criteria are kept in mind, and if careful histories and serial mental status examinations are made. Still, an occasional case of schizophrenia may begin with an affect-laden picture that resembles severe depression, and can only be diagnosed with certainty after a follow-up of several months (Chapter 6).

Course of Depression. The duration of the episode of depression prior to hospitalization among the 17 unipolar psychiatric inpatients was more prolonged than among the manics, as detailed above. The typical patient had an illness of gradual onset lasting from three to six months before admission. Commonly, a patient had failed to respond sufficiently to outpatient treatment, and a suicidal threat or attempt precipitated his admission.

The duration of index hospitalization for depression was almost exactly

---

* As mentioned (Table 2, Chapter 2) one patient not considered in this chapter qualified for both the diagnoses, depression and alcoholism, which disorders seemed to have begun at the same time.

the same as for mania. The 17 unipolar depressives were hospitalized from seven to 107 days; the modal patient was in the hospital for 27 days, and the mean was 36 days (compared to 23 and 35 days, respectively, for mania). Thirteen of the 17 unipolar depressives (76%) received ECT, a measure of the typicality and severity of the illness in these youngsters.

An assessment of outcome cannot be given until after this sample of patients has been followed up. However, as with the bipolar patients, unipolar depressives had a high incidence of readmission for the study episode. This occurred in at least seven of the 17 (41%): in three the study hospitalization itself was a readmission, and four others were readmitted to Renard for the same episode after discharge. With respect to avoidance of premature discharge, the same cautions that were discussed concerning mania also apply to depression.

Psychiatric Inpatients Who Were "Undiagnosed, Most Like Depression"

General Considerations

There were 28 subjects in our study, 14 psychiatric inpatients and 14 controls, whose disorders resembled depression more than any other syndrome, but who did not fulfill the criteria for that diagnosis. They were called "undiagnosed, most like depression." The 14 psychiatric inpatients who were so designated had a symptom picture different from that of the 14 controls. The latter failed to fulfill the criteria for depression only because of the relative mildness of their episodes, as will be shown later. The psychiatric inpatients, on the other hand, were termed "undiagnosed," because their clinical pictures were atypical. Their disorders were not mild.

The reasons for considering these 14 patients as a group were that dysphoric affect was their most prominent symptom, and that the clinical picture did not resemble any other syndrome more than it resembled depression. Only long-term follow-up and family studies can reveal whether these subjects, or some of them, should be justifiably grouped together as a clinical entity. Our prospective longitudinal study may shed light on the question of whether depression presents atypically in adolescents, then typically in the same population during adulthood. The follow-up investigation will also help determine whether the term "character neurosis" or "depressive personality disorder" may be useful in describing a sample of patients with affect-laden disorders who are neither sociopaths, hysterics, alcoholics, or drug abusers. Such terms may be legitimate if the disorders prove chronic, woven into the context of personality over a period of years without remission. It is also conceivable that an "undiagnosed, most like depression" syndrome may be a precursor of alcoholism and drug abuse, or even schizophrenia. Only time will tell. For the present, we must be content with describing the patients and their backgrounds.

Demographic and Family Data

The psychiatric inpatients who were "undiagnosed, most like depression" had the same sex distribution as those with definite depression, five boys and nine girls. But they were younger at the time of the index admission (mean 16.0 years *vs.* 17.6 years) and at the time of first onset of symptoms (14.7 *vs.* 15.9 years). Ten of the 14 had their first evidence of this disorder before they were 16 years old.

Six (21%) of the natural parents had been psychiatrically ill: there were two depressed mothers, two undiagnosed mothers, and two alcoholic fathers. This pattern does not help to distinguish the group diagnostically, since it does not differ from the family history of the typical depressives, nor from the family histories of other diagnostic subgroups among the adolescent psychiatric inpatients. Five of the 14 subjects (36%) had a least one parent with a history of psychiatric illness.

Compared with the 17 teenagers in the psychiatric hospital for typical unipolar depression, fewer of the 14 who were "undiagnosed, most like depression" were from families in the professional-executive category (zero *vs.* five), or families that earned more than $10,000 per year (four *vs.* eleven). However, the family backgrounds of the two groups were not different with regard to the amount or type of parental psychopathology, or disruption by death or divorce. The undiagnosed group had fewer subjects with I.Q.'s of 120 or higher than did the typically depressed group of psychiatric inpatients (two *vs.* seven), but the career aspirations of the undiagnosed group were just as high.

Premorbid Personality

Premorbid personality difficulties were the rule, and onset of disabling psychopathology was hard to date with certainty. Twelve of the 14 had ongoing problems such as nervousness, excessive shyness, temper outbursts, and antagonistic dealings with others before the onset of the disabling psychiatric symptoms. In addition, six of the 14 had at least the possibility of organic brain dysfunction prior to the onset of the depression-like syndrome: patient Y-003 was knocked unconscious in a fall from a chair at five months of age, and for the next three years she had breath-holding spells, turning blue with each; Y-015 had delusions of harm coincident with febrile illnesses during childhood; Y-017 had had chronic headaches since hit on the head by a baseball 4½ years before admission; Y-040 had been a hyperactive child; Y-047 had epilepsy; and Y-074 had early brain damage and mild mental retardation.

Onset, Symptoms, and Course of the Disorder

The clinical pictures of the "undiagnosed, most like depression" group cannot properly be presented as if this were a discrete syndrome like depression or mania. This was not a homogeneous group clinically, but a few general statements are warranted. First, the disorders began at a younger age (mean 14.7 years, median 15 years) than those of the typical depressives (mean 15.9, median 16). Second, the disorders usually arose in the context of pre-existing emotional symptoms and were chronic rather than episodic: nine of the 14 had been ill for more than six months, six for more than a year. Third, compared to the psychiatric inpatients with typical depression, the undiagnosed psychiatric inpatients had a lower incidence of most symptoms, but a higher incidence of crying, irritability, manipulative behavior, and antagonism toward parents. Table 23, listing the ten leading symptoms among those two groups of psychiatric inpatients, illustrates these points. Typical depressives had a greater relative prominence of hopelessness, death wishes, and vegetative symptoms, whereas among the undiagnosed subjects irritability, nervousness, and weeping were relatively more important compared to other leading symptoms. Five of the 14 undiagnosed subjects (36%) had attempted suicide, three of them within a week of admission, all five within a year. None of the 14 had a history of abusing alcohol or drugs, although eight had used alcohol to a slight degree.

TABLE 23

Leading Symptoms among Psychiatric Inpatients with Depressive Syndromes

Definite Depression N = 19*		"Undiagnosed, Most Like Depression" N = 14	
	%		%
Depressed mood, sad	95	Depressed mood, sad	79
Hopeless	89	Task disability	71
Want to die	89	Nervous	64
Task disability	89	Trouble concentrating	64
Thoughts of suicide	84	Crying†	64
Trouble concentrating	84	Thoughts of suicide	57
Loss of interest	79	Hopeless	57
Nervous	74	Loss of interest	43
Insomnia†	74	Irritability†	43
Anorexia†	74	Want to die	43

* Includes the two bipolar patients who were depressed.

† Does not appear as a leading symptom in the other group.

The duration of stay in the hospital for the index admission was less than for typical depressives (mean 24 days, *vs.* 36 days for psychiatric inpatients with depression). The median patient stayed only two weeks, half as long as the median stay for the unipolar depressives. In general, this group was not as ill as the typical depressives. As a measure of this, only 21% received ECT, compared to 76% of the latter group. Improvement was the rule, as is usually the case in psychiatric hospitalization for any disorder, but it was seldom dramatic, given the relative chronicity of the problems in most subjects. Five of the 14 patients had more than one admission to a psychiatric hospital during the index episode: two patients had two admissions, one had three, and two had four admissions.

Since the psychiatric inpatients who were "undiagnosed, most like depression" were not a homogeneous group, several case reports are necessary to illustrate clinical characteristics of this sample. In the following patient the affective disorder was preceded and accompanied by an incapacitating somatic symptom:

> Y-017—This 19-year-old white boy was six weeks premature at birth. Delivery was complicated by placenta praevia, aspiration of blood, apnea, and dehydration. As an infant he had feeding problems. In growing up he was overindulged by his parents. He became somewhat perfectionistic, did very well in school, had an I.Q. of 119. He described himself as always nervous, a "worry wart." He had occasional mild frontal headaches, beginning at an uncertain age.
>
> When he was 15 he was struck on the head by a baseball, was dazed, but not unconscious. Headaches became more severe then and never completely went away thereafter. At age 18, while he was working in a noisy asphalt plant, the symptom worsened: bifrontal, non-throbbing headaches incapacitated him at work and later in his college studies. He became increasingly nervous and irritable, unable to concentrate, and was admitted to a neurology service for 16 days, four months prior to the study admission. A complete workup, including brain scan and pneumoencephalogram failed to reveal neuropathology.
>
> After discharge he did not return to college. Nervousness increased, and he began to have crying spells accompanied by the feeling that he was letting his parents down. Because of the persistent headaches and psychiatric symptoms he was admitted to Renard Hospital.
>
> The patient himself was discouraged and irritated on admission, embarrassed about being in a psychiatric hospital. He was cooperative, but a bit demanding of indulgence. He did not appear to suffer unduly from symptoms, was treated with aspirin, and pushed to

participate in the hospital occupational and recreational programs. He improved.

The following patient demonstrated features of both hysteria and anxiety neurosis, as well as affective disorder.

Y-003—This 15-year-old white girl was knocked unconscious in a fall from her high chair at age 5 months. From then until age 3 years she had breath-holding spells during which she would turn blue and fall down.

She was outgoing, happy, and talkative till age 11, after which she was less sociable. At age 13, she began to have anxiety attacks, with palpitations, nausea, hyperventilation, tetany, and fainting. These occurred when she was in unpleasant situations or wanted to avoid activity such as the physical education class at school. At about the same time (age 13), she began to ruminate about her grandfather's having allegedly undressed her and caressed her genitalia once when she was 8 years old. She began to feel "ruined," unworthy, and deprived of her ambition to marry a minister and counsel teenagers.

Beginning at age 14, five months before admission, she spent more and more time in her room, avoiding activities with peers. She began to fear growing up, disgusted with the prospect of adult sexuality. She developed depressed moods and suicidal ruminations and said she made at least one attempt three months before admission, taking 15 to 20 aspirin tablets and not telling her parents. Accompanying these symptoms was increased irritability, rudeness to her younger siblings, and overtly manipulative behavior with her parents. By the time of her admission to the hospital for persistence of all these symptoms, the patient described herself as genuinely suffering, while the parents unsympathetically described her as selfish and play-acting.

Upon admission she expressed death wishes: "my only hope for the future is that I won't live too long," but her depressive affect seemed shallow, and at other times she was coquettish and joking.

The next case concerns a boy with long standing affective symptoms which worsened under stress:

Y-026—This 19-year-old white boy had been "mopey" and rather depressed since age 16, according to his mother, generally feeling out of place among his peers in his socially and academically prestigious prep school. At age 18, one year prior to admission, he left home for the first time to attend college. There he found himself to be "sad without a real reason," although he at times attributed it to separation from his girl friend. He described the feeling as being like a "black devil inside." He returned home after six weeks and just sat around the house. His frustration was at times manifested by temper outbursts. He saw a psychiatrist at the time, was described as "unusually tense and unhappy," and without a goal in life. For the following semester, he enrolled in a local college to escape being drafted into military service. His mood fluctuated over the next seven months before admission, and less than two weeks before admission he entered a third college close to home. Shortly thereafter, he received a letter from his girl friend saying that she was dating another boy. He became very upset, hit doors with his fists, then took 20 muscle-relaxing pills in what he described as an "attention-getting" gesture. He told his roommate and was admitted to the university infirmary, where he became unconscious for a few hours. He was transferred to Renard Hospital when medically clear. Upon admission and during his hospital stay he showed little overtly depressed affect.

The next case was that of a rather strange boy with premorbid difficulties, in whom the staff could not distinguish between atypical depression and early onset schizophrenia. There seemed to be a temporal connection between the onset of sexual feelings at puberty and his increase in behavioral problems, with incestuous and aggressive feelings toward his mother.

Y-040—This 15-year-old white boy was hyperkinetic as a child when at home, but quiet at school. He showed reluctance to attend school at age 11. This behavior recurred at age 12 for one or two months, when he used various physical complaints as transparent excuses, or simply refused to attend, throwing temper tantrums if he was coerced.

He had few friends in school but made good grades when he attended. At age 14, he abruptly told his mother he wanted to have have intercourse with her, and started to undress her. Then he broke into tears and asked her to slap him. He said in retrospect that he was angry at her before the incident. One week later he began missing school again, saying he felt badly. He gained weight and was given amphetamines by his doctor, which he was said to use sparingly. Impulsivity and irritability increased after this. At age 15, he began to try on his mother's clothes in secret and once tried to masturbate in front of her.

When he was 15½, he attended only the first week of the school's fall term, thereafter refusing to go. After a sudden inexplicable episode of rage directed at this younger brother, and destruction of furniture, he was admitted to another psychiatric hospital, and given ECT for possible depression. Upon discharge, he had more loss of interest and slovenliness, and slept a great deal. He began eating excessively. Three weeks after discharge he again received a course of ECT at the other hospital. After discharge he would not leave home, and had histrionic crying episodes. He took an overdose of aspirin in a suicide attempt. He began to have the desire to inflict pain on his brother and to pick at his own skin to make it bleed. He developed repetitive behavior, for example, saying goodnight on each of the 13 steps leading to bed and insisting on 13 replies. His temper increased, and he would put his hands around his mother's neck to choke her. He would stand before a mirror calling himself an "ugly weirdo." In the five months before the index admission he gained 40 pounds, to 210.

There was no history of drug or alcohol abuse, nor of hallucinations or delusions.

Upon admission he appeared uninterested in the interview and evasive. He was passive and did not appear especially depressed.

The following early adolescent developed psychiatric disability which was temporally related to bereavement.

Y-064—This 12-year-old white girl had an emotionally stable personality, although she was restless and moderately obese. Five months before the index admission her father, with whom she was close, died suddenly in her presence (of natural causes). The patient grieved heavily for a week, then resumed school and was well, though sad. Three months later she began to have "a funny feeling inside" and difficulty concentrating on schoolwork. She began to dream about her father and to be nervous, irritable, and depressed. She stopped going to church, saying "God did my father dirty." During the two months prior to admission, she had several unprovoked spells of enraged behavior, in which she was overtly hostile toward her mother: cursing, laughing, throwing water on her, and pinching her. She would misuse objects her mother cherished such as the family Bible and a picture of her father. Admission to the hospital was precipitated when she wrote a note, "Mom, I'm sick. I want help, but you don't want to help me."

One patient in the "undiagnosed, like depression" group had mild mental retardation and developed the insidious onset of profoundly depressed affect and incapacity, coincident with bizarre features that suggested the possibility of schizophrenia.

Y-074—This 17-year-old white boy fell from a moving car at 3½ years of age with no immediate sequelae. At age 6, he was identified as a slow learner and was in special schools thereafter. Psychologic testing at age 9 revealed full scale I.Q.'s of 73 (Stanford-Binet) and 75 (W.I.S.C.). At that time he was noted to be "immature, distractable, hyperactive, fearful," and socially withdrawn, teased by his peers for oddness and obesity.

His intellectual and social incapacity continued, increasing at age 14 when he got into a fight and was expelled from a school. Thereafter he showed some overtly depressed affect. By age 15, he developed the odd mannerism of rubbing his leg against objects.

When the patient was 16, his brother, who had helped provide him with peer contacts, left home. He withdrew further, lost interest in school, ate sporadically, and began to neglect personal hygiene. His family brought him to a psychiatric clinic, where, despite treatment with thioridazine, he remained ill. Compulsive touching of his body and other objects began, along with facial grimaces, posturing, and occasional urinary incontinence.

Two months before admission, learning that he would have to stay in a challenging work experience program, he "fell apart" according to his family. He lost further interest, appetite, and weight, and he became increasingly defiant of his parents and more slovenly. He talked of seeing "flying saucers." He felt guilty, worthless, a burden to others, and hopelessly ill. Upon admission to the hospital he said "I don't have much living in me. There are a lot of nice people here, and I feel just like a dirty rat. Some guys just don't have it. I'm not much of a human being: not very intelligent, not good looking, not much of anything. I'm like a snake pit, can't get out. I don't know what to take."

The next case presented with a hypochrondriacal preoccupation and depressed affect, but had a premorbid history of some histrionic behavior and moderate antisocial acting-out.

Y-038—This 18-year-old black girl had always done below average work in school. She had a history of some truancy, minor thefts and lying since her early teens, and she had disciplinary problems at school from smoking and occasionally fighting. However, she was never suspended. She described herself as always having been easily upset, shouting and throwing things at such times, and having blurred vision and a lump in her throat. She drank in taverns twice a week. Despite this she completed high school on schedule and worked full time during the year prior to admission.

Psychiatric disability began four months before admission, when she developed a chest cold and became obsessed with the idea that she had cancer. Negative physical examination, chest x-rays, and electrocardiograms failed to reassure her, and she repeatedly requested more examinations. Two to three months before admission, she began to have anxiety attacks, with hyperventilation and chest pain, and to become depressed and anorectic. She lost 20 pounds. Two months before admission she missed two weeks of work because she was afraid she would die if she left the house. At some time during the two months before admission she thought of suicide and once held a knife to her chest while her father was watching. She later stated that this was for the purpose of gaining attention.

On the day of admission she developed a throbbing sensation in her chest, her eyes closed partially, and she heard a voice saying "Come to me." She interpreted it as God calling her for being "evil, and drinking and going to taverns, not going to church."

In the hospital she appeared only moderately depressed at first, then became increasingly demanding and manipulative over the course of 11 days of hospitalization.

The last patient in this group was (as confirmed by 3½ year follow-up) on her way to developing a chronic illness. Her clinical picture was characterized by extreme irritability and combativeness at the time of the study. She also had a strong family history of typical affective disorder.

Y-025—This 15-year-old white girl was quiet, helpful, and affectionate until age 13, 1½ years before admission. At that time she developed respiratory infections and was hospitalized for pain in the chest. Medical workup was unremarkable, but the patient magnified her physical complaints. After this she changed markedly, and over the succeeding 20 months she became increasingly depressed and irritable. There was no history of life stress or change in the family. The patient began to quarrel, verbally abusing the family without apparent reason. Her mother became extremely solicitous, which further enraged the patient. She developed temper tantrums, cursing and tearing things up. Her concern with the possibility of physical illness increased. She also thought herself to be ugly. Concentration on academic work became a problem for the first time. She was easily fatigued and complained constantly about school. She was discouraged, cried, whined, and thought of suicide. Because of her unmanageable behavior at home she was admitted to psychiatric hospitals twice, 13 months and two months prior to index admission, treated with psychotherapy and antidepressants, but did not sustain her brief improvement.

On admission she wept copiously, said she had never been happy. She was uncooperative in the interview, blaming her parents for everything and expressing feelings of worthlessness. She felt she had lived out her life and was going to die.

The patient's mother had recurrent depressions. Her older sister had had a psychotic depression at age 19, and her maternal grandmother committed suicide in a depression. (Follow-up of this patient 3½ years later revealed a more typical course of chronic depression with irritability. The patient had had a total of five psychiatric admissions and much outpatient treatment by age 19, and never responded well to psychotherapy, antidepressants, or ECT.)

Ill Controls Who Were "Undiagnosed, Most Like Depression"

The control subjects who were labeled "undiagnosed, most like depression" failed to fulfill the criteria for typical depression only because of a paucity of symptoms. Each of them had a period of dysphoric affect during which he was different from his usual self. Eight subjects had their psychiatric disorders at the time of the study, six had had them only in the past. There was nothing in the clinical picture or course of these illnesses to distinguish them from typical depressions except their relative mildness. For example, each symptom usually appeared with less frequency than among the control subjects who fulfilled the criteria for definite depression: specific feelings of sadness appeared in 79% of the definitely depressed controls, and 64% of the controls who were "undiagnosed, most like depression." Comparable figures were, respectively: hopelessness, 57% *vs.* 21%; nervousness, 64% *vs.* 21%; loss of interest, 43% *vs.* 29%; task disability, 71% *vs.* 0%; death wishes, 43% *vs.* 29%; suicide attempts, 36% *vs.* 7%, and so on for almost all psychologic symptoms. However, the two groups had a comparable incidence of somatic symptoms, which may have been the effect of their non-psychiatric disorders.

There were five boys and nine girls among the controls who were "undiagnosed, most like depression," a typical sex distribution for affective disorder. However, at the time of their first depression-like syndromes the 14 controls were younger than had been the 25 psychiatric inpatients and eight controls with typical unipolar depression (mean 14.5 *vs.* 15.9 years). The duration of episodes was ascertainable in 11 of the 14 subjects and varied from three weeks to three years, with seven of the 11 ill for less than nine months. Two subjects had recurrent mild depressive episodes of indeterminate duration.

Like the eight typically depressed controls, the 14 subjects "undiagnosed, most like depression" had a higher incidence of psychopathology in the parents than did the psychiatrically well controls. Three fathers and one mother were alcoholics, one mother had depression, and another mother had a psychiatric illness of undetermined type. Thus six of 28 parents (22%) were ill, compared to the 9% of the parents of controls without psychiatric disorder.

In summary, it would seem legitimate to regard these 14 controls as having milder episodes of the same disorder as the eight controls with definite depression. We will discuss all 22 as a group.

Association among Medical Illness, Parental Psychopathology, and Depression in Controls

General Findings

Tables 24 and 25 illustrate a striking finding among the 22 controls with affective disorder. Among seven of the eight patients with definite depression and 13 of the 14 "undiagnosed, most like depression," onset of the psychiatric illnesses were preceded by stresses that were both objectively serious and meaningful to the patients. Only two of these subjects had ever had depressive symptoms prior to the stresses, having been previously described as moody, self-depreciating, and overly reactive. In 18 of the 20 cases with stress preceding the depressive syndromes, the patients and their families dated the onsets as immediately following the stresses; in two patients, whose depressions occurred while they were receiving steroid medication, onsets were delayed. They may, of course, have been precipitated by the steroids. In the five instances where the stresses were not continuous throughout the course of the depressions, they were nevertheless occurrences of marked significance whose psychologic impact continued long after the events themselves.

Comparison of Depressed Controls and Psychiatrically Well Controls

As discussed above, the eight controls with definite depression and the 14 "undiagnosed, most like depression" differed only with respect to severity of illness. Accordingly, we considered those 22 affectively disordered adolescents as a group and compared them to the 78 well controls with respect to demographic items and factors in the medical, social, family, and scholastic histories. They will be referred to as "depressed controls" in this section of the chapter.

The 22 depressed controls and 78 psychiatrically well controls did not differ significantly with respect to sex, race, place of residence, socio-economic background, future career goals, history of head injury, intelligence quotients, academic and disciplinary scholastic history, amount of antisocial behavior, birth order, size of sibship, bereavement experiences, history of parental divorce or separation, or duration of medical disability. The depressed controls were a mean of 17.3 years of age at the time of the study, one year older than the well controls. This may be of some importance in that they had been at risk for depression for one year longer. Only two factors markedly distinguished the depressed controls from those that were well. A significantly higher proportion of depressives had parents with histories of psychiatric disorder, and a significantly higher proportion of depressives had severe medical illnesses.

With respect to the first factor, the 22 depressives had eight mothers with a history of psychiatric illness (six depressed, one alcoholic, and one hysteric) and seven fathers (six alcoholics and one undiagnosed). Thus, 15 (34%) of the parents were ill, currently or in the past, compared with 17 (11%) of the parents of well controls, a significant difference ($p < 0.05$). Three depressed patients had both mothers and fathers with a history of psychiatric illness, whereas nine had only one ill parent. The 17 well controls with a history of parental psychopathology each had only one sick parent. So 55% of the depressed group had at least one sick parent, compared to 22% of the well group ($p < 0.01$).

With respect to the second factor, to ascertain the severity of medical disorder, it had been recorded for each control whether the probable outcome of his non-psychiatric disorder was complete recovery without defect, persistent defect without disability, chronic disability, or death. This judgment had been made independently of the knowledge of whether the patient had a psychiatric illness. Among the depressed controls, 68% had a probable outcome of chronic disability or death compared to only 37% of the well controls ($p < 0.05$). The depressed patients also differed from the well ones with respect to other indices of severity of their non-psychiatric disorders. For example, significantly more (77% *vs.* 54%, $p < 0.05$) had been hospitalized more than once for non-psychiatric illness; the currently depressed patients were in the non-psychiatric hospitals almost twice as long as the well controls, an average of 24 days *vs.* 13 days; and the parents' hopes for the patients' future, ascertained by independent questioning, had been changed for the worse by the presence of the medical illnesses in 36% of the depressed patients and 7% of those who were psychiatrically well.

TABLE 24

Relation between Stress and Affective Disorder among Controls with Definite Depression

Subject	Age and Sex	Type Stress	Interval between Onset of Stress and Onset of Affective Disorder	Was Stress Still Present at Time of Onset of Affective Disorder	Duration of Affective Disorder	Did Stress Continue for Entire Duration of Affective Disorder
C-002	18 F	Onset lupus eryth.	7 years	Yes	6 months	Yes
		Steroid treatment	6 months	Yes		Yes
C-004	19 F	None known	No stress	No stress	5 months	No stress
C-025	19 F (age 11 when depressed)	Parents separated	Immediate	Yes	9 months	Yes
C-027	15 F	Obesity	Unknown	Yes	1 year	Yes
		Moved to strange city	Immediate	Yes		No (single event)
C-032	14 M	Rheumatoid arthritis	2 years	Yes	2 months	Yes
		Steroid treatment	10 months	Yes		Yes
C-035	19 F	Childbirth by Caesarian section	Immediate	Yes	3 weeks	No (single event)
C-057	18 F	Injuries suffered in accident	Immediate	Yes	10 months	Yes
		Boy friend killed in same accident	Immediate	Yes		No (single event)
C-058	15 F	Asthma	Immediate	Yes	6 months	Yes

TABLE 25

Relation between Stress and Affective Disorder among Controls "Undiagnosed, Most Like Depression"

Subject	Age and Sex	Type Stress	Interval Between Onset of Stress and Onset of Symptoms	Was Stress Still Present at Time of Onset of Affective Disorder	Duration of Affective Disorder	Did Stress Continue for Entire Duration of Affective Disorder
C-030	19 F (14 when depressed)	Hepatitis, ulcer, missed year of school	Immediate	Yes	1–3 years	?
C-037	18 M	None known	No stress	No stress	8 months	No stress
C-038	17 F	Hodgkins disease, worsened	Hodgkins present 3½ yr., worsening occurred immediately prior to depression	Yes	3 weeks	Yes
C-040	18 F	Husband entered armed forces	Immediate	Yes	3 months	Yes
C-042	18 F	Epilepsy, rccurrence	Epilepsy present 6 months, recurrence occurred immediately prior to depression	Yes	1 month	Yes
C-043	16 F	Ulcerative colitis, recurred. "Self-depreciating all her life"	Colitis first began 6 years before, recurrence immediately prior to depression	Yes	5 months	Yes
C-046	13 F	Congenital heart disease, worsened	Disabled for 3½ years, worsening of cardiac status immediately prior to depression	Yes	4–5 months	Yes
C-051	17 M	Hodgkins disease, forced to drop school	Hodgkins present 3 years, forced to drop school immediately prior to depression	Yes	8 months	Yes
C-053	18 F (12 when first depressed)	Parents divorced (moody, easily upset "all her life" before that)	Chronic depressive symptoms worsened immediately	Yes	Episodic throughout life	No

C-070	18 F (14 when first depressed)	Encephalitis (paraplegic since then). Repair of decubiti	Immediate, worsened symptoms in association with hospitalization for decubiti	Yes	Episodic, assoc. with hospitalizations	Yes
C-086	15 F	Sarcoma	Immediate	Yes	9 months	Yes
C-096	19 M (17 when depressed)	Killed girl in auto accident	Immediate	Yes	1 year	No
C-102	19 M (17 when depressed)	Burned in accident, physical disabilities	Immediate	Yes	"several months"	Yes
C-111	19 M (15 when depressed)	Brother died	Immediate	Yes	Uncertain	No

The next question that arises concerns the nature of the association between the two factors found to be significantly more common in the depressives, parental psychopathology and severe medical disorder, and between each of these factors and the subsequent occurrence of depression. First, we discovered that the presence of both factors together strongly predicted depression in our sample of teenagers. Among the total group of adolescents considered in this paper, 50% of those with a psychiatrically ill parent and a medical prognosis of chronic disability or death developed depression, *vs.* only 9% with neither of those disadvantages ($p < 0.01$).

Next, in order to ascertain the possible independence of the two factors associated with depression, we eliminated from our calculations those patients with psychiatrically ill parents, and considered only those without parental psychopathology. We found that 23% of those with poor prognoses developed depressions, compared to 9% of those with better prognoses. Chi square corrected is 1.7, $p < 0.20$, not significant. Looking at it the other way, when we eliminated those subjects with a probable outcome of disability or death and considered only those with better prognoses, then 27% of those with parental psychopathology had depression *vs.* 9% of those without a sick parent. Chi square corrected is 1.3, $p < 0.30$, again not significant at the 5% level. Thus, from a sample of this size, we cannot say with confidence that these two factors, severe illness and parental psychopathology, operated independently of each other in their association with depression. There is an indication, however, that each may have increased our adolescents' susceptibility to affective disorder. When both factors occurred in the life of the same unfortunate youngster, the odds were 50–50 that depression would ensue, although not, it should be recalled, a depression that would require psychiatric hospitalization. In fact, only one of the depressed controls had even seen a psychiatrist as an outpatient. Table 26 illustrates the inter-

TABLE 26

Interaction among Adolescents' Medical Prognosis, Psychiatric Illness in Parents, and Depression in Adolescents

		Psychiatric Disorder in Parent: Yes	Psychiatric Disorder in Parent: No
Adolescents' Medical Prognosis	Poor	50% had depression	23% had depression
	Good	27% had depression	9% had depression

action of the two factors: having a medical illness with poor prognosis and having a psychiatrically ill parent.

Our findings are similar to Clayton's.[31, 32] In a prospective study of 109 randomly selected widows and widowers she and her co-workers found that 38 (35%) had a "depressive symptom complex" one month after the death of the spouse. Of the entire group of 109 widowed subjects, only 15% had seen or called a physician for problems related to grieving. Those with depression were not significantly more likely to request such consultation than those without depression (18% *vs.* 13%). Only one subject saw a psychiatrist, and this was at the insistence of one of the investigators.

The main difference between our findings and those of Clayton was that she found no difference between her depressed widows and non-depressed widows with respect to a family history of psychiatric disorder. One possible explanation of this may be that relatives were not interviewed in her study, whereas in 89% of our cases one parent, usually the mother, was interviewed directly.

Concerning our own findings, we do not know whether the depressive syndrome in our medically ill subjects was, in some essential way, a milder variety of the same disorder as severe depressive illness with vegetative symptoms, delusions of worthlessness, and high suicidal risk seen among psychiatric inpatients. In support of this possibility was a high incidence (34%) of psychiatric illness among the parents of our depressed patients on the non-psychiatric wards, similar to the incidence found among the parents of depressives in our psychiatric inpatient group (45%). The relative mildness of the depressions among the subjects presented in this paper does not indicate that this was essentially a different disorder from severe depressive illness, since this finding may have been artifact of selection. Severely depressed patients might have been admitted to psychiatric hospitals, not medical wards, despite the concurrence of medical disorders. The projected follow-up of our control sample and their relatives and the longitudinal comparison of their course with that of our psychiatric inpatients may provide an answer to this question.

Our other findings, that both parental psychopathology and very severe medical illness may render an adolescent susceptible to the development of depression, are in accordance with common sense and with the findings of others. First, it is well established that psychiatric disorders run in families. The nature of the possible causal link between psychiatric illness in the parents and psychiatric illness in their offspring may have been genetic, environmental, or a combination of both. We were not able to ascertain the relative importance of heredity and life experience in the depressions of our adolescent subjects.

Second, much anecdotal information over the years, as well as systematic findings of George Brown[40] and others suggest that severe stress is more likely to lead to marked mood changes than milder stress. Again, we should remember that the nature of the connection between disruptive life events and subsequent emotional turmoil has not yet been discovered, as we do not yet understand the biologic essence of depression (either the mood or the syndrome) nor many of the physiologic concomitants of depression in the brain and the rest of the body. Clinical studies alone will obviously not provide sufficient clarification of this issue.

SUMMARY

Affective Disorders in Hospitalized Teenagers

Sixty-six of the 220 subjects of this study (44 psychiatric inpatients, 22 controls) had predominantly affective syndromes. Among the 44 psychiatric inpatients with these disorders, three subgroups were considered: typical unipolar depressives, typical bipolars (who had had at least one episode of mania), and an atypical undiagnosed group who did not fulfill the criteria for depression but whose illnesses resembled depression more than any other syndrome ("undiagnosed, most like depression"). Those patients hospitalized for typical affective disorder closely resembled adults with mania and depression with respect to the clinical picture and the severity of illness. There was evidence that depression began earlier than mania and that unipolar patients had a higher incidence of premorbid emotional instability than did bipolars.

The atypical "undiagnosed" patients were characterized by premorbid psychiatric difficulties, earlier onset than typical depressives, chronicity, and more irritability and interpersonal discord. Only follow-up will determine whether some of these subjects may later be classified as a distinct syndrome, perhaps a "depressive personality disorder;" whether some are merely early onset depressives; and whether some develop other disorders, for example, alcoholism or schizophrenia.

The 22 medically hospitalized controls with affective disorder included eight with definite depression and 14 with typical, but milder, affective disturbance and too few symptoms for the research diagnosis of depression. In 20 of those 22 patients, the onset and persistence of the affective illnesses were associated with serious life stress, usually medical illness requiring great adaption on the part of the patients. Evidence is presented that disorders in the parents, especially depression and alcoholism, and the severity of the intercurrent medical illnesses were important predisposing factors in these depressions of medically ill teenagers.

REFERENCES

1. Helgason, T. Epidemiology of mental disorders in Iceland. Acta Psychiatr. Scand. *40:* (Suppl. 173) 1964.
2. Winokur, G., Clayton, P. J., and Reich, T. *Manic Depressive Illness.* St. Louis, C. V. Mosby, 1969.
3. Hudgens, R. W., de Castro, M. I., and de Zuniga, E. A. Psychiatric illness in a developing country: a clinical study. Am. J. Public Health *60:* 1788–1805, 1970.
4. Perris, C., editor. A study of bipolar (manic-depressive) and unipolar recurrent depressive psychoses. Acta Psychiatr. Scand. *42:* (Suppl. 194), 1966.
5. Kraepelin, E. *Manic-Depressive Insanity and Paranoia.* Edinburgh, E. & S. Livingstone, Ltd., 1921.
6. *DSM II: Diagnostic and Statistical Manual of Mental Disorders,* Ed. 2. Washington, American Psychiatric Association, 1968.
7. Grinker, R. R., Sr., Miller, J., Sabshin, M., Nunn, R., and Nunnally, J. C. *The Phenomena of Depressions.* New York, Paul B. Hoeber, Inc., 1961.
8. Lange, J. "Die Endogenen und Reaktiven Gemütserkrankungen," cited in Bumke, O. *Handbuch der Geisteskrankheiten.* Berlin, J. Springer, 1928.
9. Robins, E., and Guze, S. B. Classification of affective disorders: the primary-secondary, the endogenous-reactive, and the neurotic-psychotic concepts. In *Recent Advances in the Psychobiology of the Depressive Illnesses: Proceedings of a Workshop Sponsored by the National Institute of Mental Health,* Williams, T. A., Katz, M. M. and Shield, J. A., Jr., Eds. (pp. 283–293). U.S. Government Printing Office, 1971.
10. Hall, G. S. *Adolescence, Its Psychology and Its Relations to Physiology, Anthropology, Sociology, Sex, Crime, Religion and Education.* New York and London, D. Appleton, 1904.
11. Wille. Die Psychosen der Pubertätsalters. Leipzig, 1898 (cited in reference #10).
12. Kasinin, J., and Kaufman. The functional psychoses in childhood. Am. J. Psychiatry *9:* 307–384, 1929.
13. Kasinin, J. The affective psychoses in children. Am. J. Psychiatry *10:* 897–926, 1930.
14. Despert, J. L. Suicide and depression in children. Nerv. Child *9:* 378–389, 1952.
15. Harms, E. Differential pattern of manic-depressive disease in childhood. Nerv. Child *9:* 326–356, 1952.
16. Campbell, J. Manic-depressive psychoses in children: report of 18 cases. J. Nerv. Ment. Dis. *116:* 424–439, 1952.
17. Campbell, J. D. *Manic-Depressive Disease.* Philadelphia, J. B. Lippincott Co., 1953.
18. Sands, D. E. The psychoses of adolescence. J. Ment. Sci. *102:* 308–316, 1956.
19. Landolt, A. D. Follow-up studies on circular manic-depressive reactions occurring in the young. Bull. NY Acad. Med. *33:* 65, 1957.
20. Olsen, T. Follow-up study of manic-depressive patients whose first attack occurred before the age of 19. Acta Psychiatr. Scand (Suppl. 162). *37:* 45–51, 1961.
21. Anthony, J., and Scott, P. Manic-depressive psychosis in childhood. Child Psychol. and Psychiatry *1:* 53–72, 1960.
22. Carter, A. B. The prognostic factors of adolescent psychosis. J. Ment. Sci. *88:* 31–81, 1942.
23. Toolan, J. M. Depression in children and adolescents. Am. J. Orthopsychiatry *32:* 404–415, 1962.
24. Frommer, E. Depressive illness in childhood. Br. Med. J. *2:* 117–136, 1968.
25. Poznanski, E., and Zrull, J. P. Childhood depression. Arch. Gen. Psychiatry *23:* 8–15, 1970.
26. King, L. J., and Pittman, G. D. A six year follow-up study of sixty-five adolescent

patients: predictive value of presenting clinical picture. Br. J. Psychiatry *115:* 1437–1441, 1969.

27. Annesley, P. T. Psychiatric illness in adolescence: presentation and prognosis. J. Ment. Sci. *107:* 268–278, 1961.
28. Weiner, I. B. *Psychological Disturbance in Adolescence.* New York, John Wiley & Sons, 1970.
29. Masterson, J. F., Jr. *The Psychiatric Dilemma of Adolescence.* Boston, Little, Brown and Co., 1967.
30. Kendell, R. E., Cooper, J. E., Gourlay, A. J., Copeland, J. R. M., Sharpe, L., and Gurland, B. J. Diagnostic criteria of American and British psychiatrists. Arch. Gen. Psychiatry *25:* 123–130, 1971.
31. Clayton, P. J., Halikas, J. A., and Maurice, W. L. The bereavement of the widowed. Dis. Nerv. Syst., *32:* 597–604, 1971.
32. Clayton, P. J., Halikas, J. A., and Maurice, W. L. The depression of widowhood. Br. J. Psychiatry *120:* 71–77, 1972.
33. Clayton, P. J., Halikas, J. A., Maurice, W. L., and Robins, E. Anticipatory grief and widowhood. Br. J. Psychiatry *122:* 47–51, 1973.
34. Hudgens, R. W., Morrison, J. R., and Barchha, R. G. Life events and onset of primary affective disorders. Arch. Gen. Psychiatry *16:* 134–145, 1967.
35. Hudgens, R. W., Robins, E., and DeLong, W. B. The reporting of recent stress in the lives of psychiatric patients. Br. J. Psychiatry *117:* 635–643, 1970.
36. Morrison, J. R., Hudgens, R. W., and Barchha, R. G. Life events and psychiatric illness. Br. J. Psychiatry *114:* 423–432, 1968.
37. Birley, J. L. T., and Brown, G. W. Crises and life changes preceding the onset or relapse of acute schizophrenia: clinical aspects. Br. J. Psychiatry *116:* 327–333, 1970.
38. Brown, G. W., and Birley, J. L. T. Crises and life changes and the onset of schizophrenia. J. Health Soc. Behav. *9:* 203–214, 1968.
39. Brown, G. W. Life events and psychiatric illness: some thoughts on methodology and causality. J. Psychosom. Res. *16:* 311–320, 1972.
40. Brown, G. W., Sklair, F., Harris, T. O., and Birley, J. L. T. Life events and psychiatric disorders. Part I: Some methodological issues. Psychol. Med. *3:* 74–87, 1973.
41. Brown, G. W., Harris, T. O., and Peto, J. Life events and psychiatric disorders. Part II: Nature of causal link. Psychol. Med. (in press).
42. Paykel, E. S., Myers, J. K., Dienett, M. N., Klerman, G. L., Lindenthal, J. J., and Pepper, M. P. Life events and depression: a controlled study. Arch. Gen. Psychiatry *21:* 753–760, 1969.
43. Paykel, E. S., Prusoff, B. A., and Ulenhuth, E. H. Scaling of life events. Arch. Gen. Psychiatry *25:* 340–347, 1971.
44. Holmes, T. H., and Rahe, R. H. The social readjustment rating scale. J. Psychosom. Res. *2:* 213–218, 1967.
45. Holmes, T. H., and Masuda, M. Life change and illness susceptibility. Presented at "Symposium on Separation and Depression: Clinical and Research Aspects," at the annual meeting of the American Association for the Advancement of Science, Chicago, Illinois, December 26–30, 1970 (in press).
46. Cassidy, W. L., Flanagan, N. B., Spellman, M., and Cohen, M. E. Clinical observations in manic-depressive disease, a quantitative study of one hundred manic-depressive patients and fifty medically sick controls. JAMA *164:* 1536–1546, 1957.
47. Welner, J., and Strömgren, E. Clinical and genetic studies on benign schizophreniform psychoses based on a follow-up. Acta Psychiatr. Neurol. Scand. *33:* 377–399, 1958.

48. Clayton, P. J., Rodin, L. and Winokur, G. Family History Studies: III. Schizo-affective disorder, clinical and genetic factors, including a one to two year follow-up. Compr. Psychiatry *9:* 31–49, 1968.

49. Woodruff, R. A., Jr., Murphy, G. E., and Herjanic, M. The natural history of affective disorder: 1. Symptoms of 72 patients at the time of index hospital admission. J. Psychiatr. Res. *5:* 255–263, 1967.

5

Suicide communications and attempts

PSYCHIATRIC ILLNESS AND SUICIDAL BEHAVIOR

In the United States the "typical" suicide is a white man, middle-aged or older, suffering from depressive disorder or chronic alcoholism. If he is an alcoholic, according to Murphy and Robins,[1] the timing of his death may make sense in terms of recent devastating circumstances (loss of job, separation from spouse, etc.) which are consequences of his long-standing illness. If he has primary depression, his suicide may seem logical only in the context of the disordered judgment and pathologically lowered self-esteem that so often mark the depressive syndrome: "I'm rotten. My family will do better if I'm dead." Such remarks may bear no resemblance to the truth, and the man's suicide may make little sense to the outside observer.

Suicide rarely, if ever, occurs among the psychiatrically well in this country, and its incidence among people who are hopelessly ill with medical disorders is surprisingly low.[2] The popular press often attributes suicides to specific life circumstances, but systematic studies bear out that serious psychiatric illness is almost always a necessary precondition for self-destruction, even when objectively stressful circumstances have triggered the act itself.

The typical suicide *attempter* is a young woman or an adolescent. The role of psychiatric illness among attempters is less clear than among successful suicides, especially in the younger age groups. Certainly hysterics, sociopaths, and drug abusers, as well as depressives and alcoholics, appear in large numbers among the attempters.[3] And the busy emergency room physician, after pumping out the stomach of yet another teenage girl who has impulsively taken too much aspirin following a lover's quarrel, may question whether such suicide attempters are really sick by any reasonable definition of the word.

There are many exceptions to the above generalizations, of course. Many older men are unsuccessful in their attempts to kill themselves, and some young women and adolescents commit suicide. Studies have established that suicide attempters and completers form two distinct but overlapping populations.[4] Although estimates vary, about 25% of suicides are known to have made previous attempts,[5, 6] and between 10 and 15% of unsuccessful attempters later succeed in killing themselves.[7]

SUICIDAL COMMUNICATION AND BEHAVIOR AMONG ADOLESCENTS: GENERAL CONSIDERATIONS

Not many teenagers commit suicide—744 under age 20 in the United States in 1964—but suicide was the fifth leading cause of death among adolescents that year, and there is evidence that the rate may be rising among American youth.[8] A teenager's suicide seems especially tragic, because his life has so recently begun, and because he may suffer from a curable illness of acute onset, for example, depression, not a chronic personality disorder nor a hopeless mental or physical illness.

Suicide attempts, on the other hand, seem much more prevalent among teenagers than adults. The ratio of attempts to completions is about 8:1 in adults, and has been estimated as high as 50:1 or 100:1 in adolescents.[9] There is also indirect evidence that this phenomenon has increased among the youth of this country during the past decade or so. The increase may be real, or it may only be an apparent increase, resulting from better reporting and the popularity of suicide as a topic of research and as a target for preventive measures in the mental health field. In any case, suicidal talk and action of various degrees of seriousness are major precipitants of psychiatric hospitalization for American teenagers, and an adolescent inpatient sample provides an opportunity for studying these phenomena. Of the psychiatric inpatients in our investigation, 40% had made suicide attempts. Among adults admitted to Renard Hospital, only 10 to 15% have a history of suicide attempts.[10, 11]

A number of questions about suicidal behavior, especially among adolescents, need investigation. First, what is the nature of the relationship between suicidal communications (including attempts) and completed suicide? Under what circumstances is the one predictably followed by the other? What is the relationship between psychiatric illness and suicidal behavior, or between each specific psychiatric syndrome and such communication or action? What is the prognostic significance of suicidal communication and behavior among the young? What, if any, aspects of these phenomena predict future suicidal acts, social maladjustment, or specific psychiatric disorders? How should the physician evaluate and manage the teenager who talks or acts in suicidal fashion? And finally, how can suicide be prevented, despite the limitations of our present knowledge about psychiatric illness and self-destructive tendencies? These questions will be addressed in the current chapter and in Chapter 9. More complete answers, however, should be forthcoming after our adolescent sample is followed up in adulthood.

SUICIDAL COMMUNICATION AMONG STUDY SUBJECTS

Incidence and Types of Communication among Adolescents and Adults

All 220 subjects were asked about suicide attempts (defined as ingestion or self-injury carried out by an adolescent with the stated intent to kill himself) and the timing, method, and circumstances of each such act. In addition, the last 60 of the 110 psychiatric inpatients we interviewed, and all 110 controls, were questioned as to the presence or absence at any time of the 15 specified types of suicidal communication shown in a previous study to be those most frequently expressed by psychiatric inpatients.[10] With respect to each communication we asked about timing, frequency, associated stress, concurrent psychiatric symptoms, and the identity of the person(s) to whom the patient made his statement. In this portion of the interview, an actual suicide attempt was considered one type of communication, even if the patient had told no one about it at the time of the attempt. We chose to study communications of suicidal intent rather than mere suicidal thoughts, since we wanted data comparable to those gathered from a psychiatric hospital population in a previous study, and since reported communications about suicide are potentially verifiable, whereas thoughts are not.

For purposes of studying suicidal communications, we matched the 60 psychiatric inpatients who were questioned about these phenomena with 60 of the controls for age, sex, and race. They differed little from the total study sample, having a mean age of 16.5 years, a girl: boy ratio of 57:43%, and a white: black ratio of 88:12%. Their distribution among diagnostic groups was also representative of the total sample. Among the 60 controls who were selected to match the 60 psychiatric inpatients, 37% had a psychiatric disorder.

In Table 27, three subgroups of our teenage sample (60 psychiatric inpatients, 22 psychiatrically ill controls, and 38 psychiatrically well controls) are compared with 81 adult patients. The latter subjects were all those over 19 years of age from an earlier study (DeLong and Robins[10]) of representative admissions to Renard Hospital in 1959, who had been examined with the same suicide communication protocols as our adolescents. Their mean age was 47 years (range 21 to 75); 32% were men, 68% women.

It can be seen from Table 27 that 40 (67%) of the adolescent psychiatric inpatient sample and eight (13%) of the adolescent controls had communicated suicidal intent at some time in their lives. The controls who

TABLE 27
*Types of Communication of Suicidal Intent**

	Adult Psychiatr. Patients[10] N = 81		Adolescent Psychiatr. Inpatients N = 60		Adolescent Controls		
					with Psychiatr. Illness N = 22		without Psychiatr. Illness N = 38
	%		%		%		%
1. Desire to die	37		45		27	$p < 0.01$	0
2. "Better off dead"	40		40		27	$p < 0.01$	0
3. "Family would be better off"	38		23		18	$p < 0.05$	0
4. Intent to commit suicide	35		50		27	$p < 0.01$	0
5. *Actual* suicide attempt	14	$p < 0.001$	43	$p < 0.001$	5		0
6. Reference to method	25		23	$p < 0.05$	5		0
7. Dire predictions	11		10	$p < 0.05$	0		0
8. Reference to dying before relative	16		2		0		0
9. Putting affairs in order	6		2		0		0
10. "Can't take it any longer"	21		12	$p < 0.01$	0		0
11. Reference to burial or grave	7		3		5		0
12. Afraid (or not afraid) to die	19		10	$p < 0.05$	0		0
13. Talk of others' suicides	4		8	$p < 0.05$	0		0
14. Insist family not buy new things	1		2		5		0
15. Taunts and threats	7		12		5		0
16. Other	1	$p < 0.001$	17	$p < 0.001$	0		0
Any type communication	68		67	$p < 0.05$	36	$p < 0.01$	0

* All significant differences between groups in adjacent columns are indicated in the table.

communicated intent all had psychiatric disorders. Such communications had not occurred among the well controls, but 35% of the psychiatrically ill controls had made communications.

The proportion of adolescent psychiatric patients communicating suicidal intent was the same as the proportion of adult communicators in the earlier study. Considering specific types of communication, it was only with respect to the incidence of actual suicide attempts that the adolescent patients differed significantly from the adults. This difference was striking, and there are several possible explanations for it.

First, it has been demonstrated that in the general population suicide attempts are more common among young people than among middle-aged adults. Few of the subjects in the adult comparison sample had been ill during their teens; so our adolescents were psychiatrically ill at a time in their lives when they were at a greater risk for attempts. Second, the rate of suicide attempts may have been rising in teenagers during recent years. In a review of 12 systematic studies of attempted suicides, Murphy[12] found a general rise since 1927 in the proportion of attempters under age 20, with a marked rise after 1960. In six studies of suicide attempters from 1927 to 1958, 8% of 8,499 attempters were under 20, as compared with 20.6% of the 2,426 attempters in six studies done since 1960. Third, physicians may be more likely to admit an adolescent than an adult who has made a suicide attempt, simply because he is a minor. For example, a much higher proportion (85%) of adult attempters in the comparison sample (DeLong and Robins[10]) had depression than did adolescent attempters. This suggests that the younger group of attempters may have been less serious risks for completed suicide than the older group of attempters, since depression is by far the most frequent disorder among suicides, and the physicians admitting patients to Renard Hospital know this. Thus, they may be more inclined to admit teenage attempters, even when they are not considered serious risks.

The psychiatrically ill adolescent controls, in the hospital for medical or surgical disorders, communicated suicide intent significantly less frequently than the adults or teenagers who were psychiatric inpatients. This was to be expected, since a selection criterion for controls (they must never have been hospitalized for psychiatric disorder), made it likely that even if they had a psychiatric disorder they would be less sick than the psychiatric inpatients.

Considering all the communicating subjects together, adults and teenagers, the first five types of communication listed in Table 27 were the principal ways of expressing suicidal intent. At least one of those five methods was employed by 78% of the adult communicators, and 98% of the adolescent communicators. Only 12% of the adolescent psychiatric patients was said to have used suicidal communications in a taunting, manipulative way, and those few patients also made other types of communication, which were considered to be serious.

When the adolescents who attempted suicide were compared with those who communicated intent but did not make attempts, it was found that the two groups did not differ significantly with respect to the proportion expressing any of the verbal types of communication.

Timing and Frequency of Suicidal Communications; and Persons to Whom Communications Were Made

The 48 adolescent suicide communicators may be considered as a group with respect to the frequency and timing of communication and their relationship to persons to whom suicidal intent was communicated, since the 40 psychiatric inpatients did not differ from the eight psychiatrically ill controls regarding those factors. Sixteen of the 48 "communicating" subjects (33%) first communicated suicidal intent more than one year before admission, and eight (17%) communicated such intent for the first time during the month prior to admission. The most recent communication was within the week before admission for 58% of the communicators, and within one month for 81%. During the current episode of psychiatric illness, communication was reported to have occurred at least once a week for 44% of the 48 communicators, at least once a month for 71%.

Eighty-three percent of the 48 communicators expressed suicidal intentions to at least their parents or spouses, 42% to at least other relatives or friends, and only 15% to professional persons (physicians, teachers, and counselors).

When we interviewed relatives, we identified 18% more communicators than we would have identified if only the patients had been questioned.

Factors Associated with Suicidal Communication among Psychiatric Inpatients

Among the adolescent psychiatric inpatients, suicide communicators were compared with non-communicators with respect to a variety of factors (Table 28). Of the factors listed, communicators differed significantly from non-communicators only with respect to a history of prior psychiatric hospitalization. This may only mean that communicators were more likely to have been previously hospitalized simply because they were communicators.

A depressive syndrome, definite depression or "undiagnosed, most like depression," was associated with a higher proportion of suicidal expression, although this was not significant at the 5% level. This lack of significance is attributable to the fact that many of the adolescents with syndromes other than depression nevertheless showed affective symptoms, including talk of suicide. However, there was a significant association between definite depression and actual suicide *attempts,* as will be discussed later in this chapter.

Suicidal communications in general were not predictable by sex, current age, age of first onset of psychiatric illness, duration of illness, alcohol or drug abuse, family history of psychiatric illness or suicide, loss of parent by death, or socioeconomic status of the family.

Controls Who Communicated Suicidal Intent

Eight of the 60 controls (13%) had communicated suicidal intent, and only one of them had attempted suicide.* These eight were among the 22

* Of the 50 controls who were *not* matched with the 60 psychiatric inpatients whom

TABLE 28

Comparison of Adolescent Suicide Communicators with Non-communicators
(Psychiatric Inpatients Only)

	Suicide Communicators N = 40		Non-communicators N = 20
	%		%
Proportion who were females	48		40
Proportion age 16 or younger	38		50
Mean age (years)	16.8		16.0
Age of onset, first psychiatric illness ≤ 14	43		47
Mean age of onset, first psychiatric illness (years)	14.3		13.8
Previous hospitalization for psychiatric illness	48	$p < 0.05$	20
Current episode > one year's duration	40		40
Alcohol or drug abuse	18		15
Depressive syndrome*	35		20
Hospitalization more than once for non-psychiatric illness	30		35
Psychiatric illness in primary relative	53		60
Any relative hospitalized for psychiatric illness	40		45
Family history of suicide	5		15
Natural parent died	12		5
Family of professional-managerial class	35		50
Socioeconomic index[13] of father ≥ 50 (when known)	47		62

* Definite depression or "undiagnosed, most like depression."

controls with psychiatric illness. The numbers were rather small for meaningful analysis, and there were no significant differences between communicating and non-communicating controls with respect to factors listed in Table 28. However, we also compared the communicating and non-communicating controls as to duration of their medical or surgical disorders and as to prognosis of those (non-psychiatric) illnesses. Seven of the eight communicating controls (88%) had an illness of at least six months' duration *vs.* 58% of the 52 non-communicators, a difference that is significant ($p < 0.05$). Judging by the type of medical or surgical disorder (see Chapter 4), six of the eight communicators (75%) *vs.* only 39% of noncommunicating controls, had a prognosis of chronic disability or death, a difference also significant at <0.05. Duration and severity of the medical disorder thus may have influenced suicidal symptoms. This is not surprising, since as shown in Chapter 4, the severity of a medical illness apparently predisposed our teenage control subjects to the development of a depressive syndrome.

---

we questioned about communication of suicidal intent, five (10%) had made such communications, and none had attempted suicide.

THE SUICIDE ATTEMPTERS

General Considerations

In our study the investigation of actual suicide attempts was more extensive than the investigation of other types of suicidal communication, since *all* the subjects and informants were asked about self-destructive acts (at any time in their lives) and the timing and circumstances of such acts. Forty-four (40%) of the 110 psychiatric inpatients and one control subject had attempted suicide, that is, ingested drugs or injured themselves and stated at the time or later that they had intended to die. This section of the chapter will discuss those attempters.

Influence of Depressive Illness and Female Sex on Incidence of Attempts

What were the characteristics of the adolescent suicide attempters? First, and most important, they were all psychiatrically ill, and their designation as ill did not depend upon the fact that they had attempted suicide. Psychiatrically well controls had not tried to kill themselves. Second, attempts occurred among more seriously ill subjects: only one of the 39 psychiatrically ill controls (a less sick group than the psychiatric inpatients) had tried this. Third, the attempters were predominantly girls, and the proportion of girls was highest among patients who made attempts very early in adolescence. Fourth, attempts were most likely to have occurred in the course of illnesses in which depressive affect was prominent, regardless of whether the attempter was a girl or a boy; and the more typically depressive the syndrome, the more likely it was that suicidal behavior had occurred.

Table 29 illustrates the last two points in part. (The only control who had attempted suicide, an 18-year-old girl with chronic orthopedic problems who was "undiagnosed, most like depression" is excluded from consideration here.) Forty-nine percent of the female psychiatric patients and 27% of the males had made at least one attempt ($p < 0.05$).

Thirteen (68%) of the 19 definite depressives among the psychiatric inpatients had tried to kill themselves, compared to 31 (35%) of the other 91 patients (χ^2 corrected $= 6.36$, $p < 0.02$). The diagnosis of typical depression in a teenager did not depend on the fact that a suicide attempt had occurred.

In 12 of the 15 attempters who were "undiagnosed, unclassified," depressive illness was considered one of the possible diagnoses. Their illnesses were not designated depression, because they were atypical; and they were not called "undiagnosed, most like depression," because in each case the clinical picture suggested that another syndrome (*e.g.*, antisocial

TABLE 29

Principal Diagnoses by Sex among Psychiatric Inpatients Who Attempted Suicide

	Girl Attempters N = 32	Girl Non-attempters N = 34	Boy Attempters N = 12	Boy Non-Attempters N = 32
Depression	7	2	6	4
Undiagnosed, most like depression	4	5	1	4
Undiagnosed, unclassified	12	6	3	8
Undiagnosed, optionally classified as either depression or other	1	1	0	0
Undiagnosed, most like hysteria	2	0	0	0
Antisocial personality	2	1	1	3
Undiagnosed, most like antisocial personality	2	3	0	2
Schizophrenia	1	3	0	2
Undiagnosed, most like schizophrenia	0	0	1	0
Undiagnosed, "schizoaffective"	1	4	0	2
Mania	0	6	0	5
Alcoholism	0	0	0	1
Organic brain syndrome	0	1	0	0
Mental deficiency	0	0	0	1
Anorexia nervosa	0	1	0	0
No psychiatric illness	0	1	0	0

personality, hysteria, drug abuse) should be considered as seriously as depression.

Suicide attempts were rare in mania, schizoaffective illness, schizophrenia, and "undiagnosed, like schizophrenia." Only three of the 25 psychiatric inpatients with those diagnoses had ever tried to kill themselves, and one of these (the only schizoaffective attempter) had done so during a prior episode of depression, not during his current schizoaffective illness. This is an important finding, considered together with the fact that there was such a high incidence of attempts among typical depressives. It demonstrated that among the "psychotic" subjects, those who had departed furthest from reason and whose thinking and perception were most disordered, actual suicidal behavior was unusual unless the psychosis was depression.

Type of psychiatric illness and sex distribution were thus the key factors which distinguished suicide attempters from nonattempters. These and other factors were explored further in order to characterize the attempters more completely.

Relationship between Age and Suicide Attempts

When the data were analyzed with respect to age, two main findings emerged. First, girls with undiagnosed psychiatric illness were overrepresented among the youngest (age 12 to 15) suicide attempters. There were 12 attempters who were 12 to 15 at the time of our study and five additional attempters who, although over 15 years old, had made their first suicide attempt between ages 12 and 15. Of these 17 youngest attempters, 14 were undiagnosed and 15 were girls. The diagnostic groupings were: "undiagnosed, unclassified," 7; "undiagnosed, most like depression," 5; and one each with depression, schizophrenia, antisocial personality, "undiagnosed, most like hysteria," and "undiagnosed, most like antisocial personality." Of the 17 patients who first attempted suicide by age 15, 88% were girls; but of 50 non-attempters who had been psychiatrically ill by that age (and therefore at risk for suicide attempts), only 54% were girls ($p < 0.01$). Of the 17 young attempters, then, 82% were undiagnosed; but of 45 non-attempters whose illnesses began by age 15, only 58% were undiagnosed ($p = <0.05$). Thus if a very young adolescent attempted suicide, she was most likely to be a girl with an atypical psychiatric disorder. This was true despite the fact that neither girls, nor undiagnosed patients, nor suicide attempters were overrepresented in the younger age group.

Second, adolescent suicide attempters with typical depression were clustered in the older age group (17 to 19). Eleven of the 13 depressed attempters were 17 or older. Among the 29 suicide attempters age 17 to 19, 38% had definite depression (*vs.* 17% of the entire psychiatric inpatient sample who were definite depressives). This age distribution is explained by the fact that the total sample of depressives also clustered in the older age group, whether or not they were suicide attempters, and regardless of sex.

Psychiatric Illness in Parents of Attempters

Considering only the 110 psychiatric inpatients, a greater proportion of the parents of the 44 suicide attempters had a history of psychiatric illness than did the parents of the 66 non-attempters. Among the attempters, 44% of the fathers and 31% of the mothers were ill; among non-attempters, the respective figures were 23% and 18%. Fifty-seven percent of attempters and 39% of non-attempters had at least one sick parent (not significant). The difference was accounted for by the fact that girl attempters (who comprised 73% of the suicide-attempting group) had a strikingly high proportion of sick fathers (57%) and more than their share of sick mothers (33%). Two-thirds of their sick fathers were alcoholics, whereas half their ill mothers were "undiagnosed"—the predominant disorders among those parents (and the only disorders which were more prominent among the parents of attempters than of non-attempters). Boy attempters and non-attempters did not differ with respect to incidence of parental psychopathology.

Interestingly, only 9% of suicide attempters had a family history of suicide *vs.* 16% of non-attempters (N.S.).

Relationship between Sex and Diagnosis among Attempters

Table 28 illustrates that 50% of the boys who attempted suicide had typical depression *vs.* 22% of the girls who made attempts (not significant). The girl attempters were distributed among more diagnostic groups and included more patients with behavioral problems, for example, those with traits of antisocial personality or hysteria, and several of those in the "undiagnosed, unclassified" group. This accounted for our finding that academic and discipline problems, as well as negative attitudes toward parents, were more common among girl attempters than among boy attempters, although in the psychiatric inpatient sample as a whole such problems were more prevalent among boys than girls. In view of this fact, and the increased prevalence of alcoholism among the fathers of girls who attempted suicide, it was not surprising to also find that more girl attempters than boy attempters had parents with socially deviant behavior—jail, drunkenness, unstable employment records, and divorce.

Duration of Illness and Suicide Attempts

Suicide attempters and non-attempters did not differ significantly with respect to duration of psychiatric illness. An insignificantly greater proportion of non-attempters than attempters (30% *vs.* 18%) had been sick less than three months with the current episode of illness. This was accounted for by the fact that fewer girl attempters (a more diagnostically heterogeneous group than by attempters) were in the acutely ill group. In fact, the average girl attempter had had the first onset of her principal psychiatric disorder three years before the index admission, whereas the average boy attempter had first been ill two years before admission.

Prior Hospitalization and Suicide Attempts

A history of prior hospitalization did not predict a suicide attempt. On the contrary, such a history was lower for both boy and girl attempters (25% and 42%, respectively) than for boys and girls as a whole (30% and 65%). This apparent paradox is explained by the fact that 68% of all attempters had tried suicide only once, thus were not repeatedly hospitalized for such behavior. In addition, the manic and schizophrenic groups, containing the highest proportion of subjects who had been previously hospitalized (59% of the 17 patients in those categories), had a very low proportion of suicide attempters (6%).

Miscellaneous Factors

More attempters (32% of those tested) than non-attempters (11%) had intelligence quotients above 120 (N.S.). This difference is accounted for by the fact that there were more typical depressives in the highly intelligent group. Some factors which did not differentiate attempters from non-attempters, even when we controlled for sex in the analysis of data were: religion, occupation of family wage earner, family income, loss of a parent or sibling through death, incidence of heterosexual or homosexual intercourse, and drug or alcohol abuse.

THE SUICIDE ATTEMPTS

General Considerations

Suicide attempts only occurred in the psychiatrically ill subjects of our study, and they only occurred at time of illness. Although this was frequently the most striking symptom in the course of a patient's illness and often precipitated a request for psychiatric care, it was rarely a common symptom for any one patient. Suicide attempts among our patients were usually psychologically serious but rarely medically serious. It was most striking that, viewed in the total context of an adolescent's illness, the attempt seldom seemed of predominant importance compared to other features of the illness, despite its often dramatic quality.

Number of Attempts and Methods Used

Of the 45 patients who had ever attempted suicide, 30 had done so once, 10 twice, three three times, one four times, and one had attempted suicide approximately 18 times. Ingestion of drugs was the method of the most recent attempt in 88% of the attempters. Preparations containing aspirin were the favored substances, probably because of their availability, and were used in almost half the cases. Over-the-counter sleeping medications and miscellaneous prescribed drugs (especially barbiturates and tranquilizers) were used with about equal frequency in the remainder of ingestion attempts. The second most popular method, stabbing or cutting (usually the wrists), was used in only 7% of the most recent attempts.

Age, Frequency and Timing of Attempts

The average attempter was 16.9 years old at the time of our study and had first become psychiatrically ill at 14.2 years of age. So, despite a mean of 2.7 years since the first onset of his illness, the average attempter had tried to kill himself only once or twice: it was a rare event in his life.

Although 40% of the patients who attempted suicide had developed their principal psychiatric illness by age 13, only 11% of them had tried

TABLE 30

Age of Onset of Principal Psychiatric Disorder and Age of First Suicide Attempt for 45 Attempters

Age	Age of Onset	Age of First Attempt
Younger than 10 years	2	0
10	2	0
11	0	0
12	7	4
13	7	1
14	3	6
15	7	6
16	8	6
17	5	11
18	2	7
19	2	4
	—	—
Total	45	45
Mean	14.2 years	16.0 years

suicide by that time (Table 30). Only 28% of those who were first sick before their 14th birthday, and who would ever attempt to kill themselves, had done so before that age. The average attempter became ill at age 14.2 years, first tried suicide almost two years later, and had his current admission to Renard Hospital one year after that first attempt. Suicide attempts did not occur before age 12 in any of our subjects.

The time of the *most recent* suicide attempt was within one week of the index admission for 36% of attempters and within a month for an additional 15%, but was more than a year before the index admission for 27%. It is of interest that 14 (31%) of the 45 patients had made their attempts without having any psychiatric care-seeking associated with their actions and without telling about them until much later. Only at the time of the index admissions, which in those cases were unrelated to the suicide attempts, did information about those early attempts emerge. These 14 patients did not differ from the total group of attempters with respect to age, sex, or diagnosis.

Motivation and Circumstances of Attempts

Compared to other psychiatric symptoms, suicide attempts are in a somewhat special category, since they are voluntary acts which may spring from other, involuntary symptoms of illness, such as low mood, poor judgment, delusions, impulsivity, and so forth. Obviously, merely having a psychiatric illness is not a sufficient precondition for a suicide attempt. Before he tries to kill himself a patient must make a decision to do so, however precipitous, misguided, or maladaptive that decision may be. In questioning our patients, we asked about their specific motives, the social and interpersonal setting of each attempt, and the sequence of events leading to the action. If an attempt had been very recent, it was usually possible to elicit such a specific account. This account gave important clues to the nature of the conflicts, interpersonal and intrapsychic, which were most troubling to the patient, and helped the doctor make decisions about diagnosis and treatment. But if a suicide attempt had occurred in the remote past, it was often impossible for a patient to describe the psychosocial context in which it had taken place. Even in telling of recent attempts, the teenager was sometimes unable or unwilling to "make it make sense" to the interviewer that he wanted to die. Whatever his diagnosis, and however distorted his judgment, the adolescent's retrospective view of a suicide attempt was at times altered by subsequent circumstances, such as increased parental concern and the complex events of psychiatric hospitalization.

The specific circumstances of suicidal acts were discovered for some or all the attempts of 32 of the 45 (44 psychiatric inpatients and one sick control) who tried to kill themselves. The impressive fact was that, whatever the apparent precipitating events of an attempt, the *basic context* in which it took place was always an ongoing psychiatric illness. The illness made it very likely, in the first place, that the adolescent would be involved in interpersonal or internal stress; and, in the second place, made it likely that he would be unduly susceptible to that stress and react with grief, anger, and death wishes.

As mentioned in Chapter 3, psychiatric illness often engendered conflict between the teenagers and their families. So it is not surprising that the leading precipitant of a suicidal attempt, occurring in at least 13 cases, was an argument with one or both parents. In eight other cases, the patient had conflict with a girlfriend, boyfriend, or spouse just before the attempt, and in two of those there were feelings of guilt concerning recent sexual intercourse. Six other precipitating events were situations of embarrassment or failure in a peer-group or school situation. Two patients tried suicide at times of special frustration with medical illness and procedures; one patient was confronted with legal difficulties over antisocial behavior; one attempted suicide on two occasions while she was intoxicated.

Among the above 32 patients and the remaining 13 for whose attempts the specific social situations were not discovered, the basic mood behind the suicidal act was depression or anger, or a mixture of both. A feeling of rejection, or frustration and helplessness, commonly followed the precipitating events. Under those circumstances, suicide seemed to the patient the only alternative, at least temporarily. All of the attempting subjects said they had wanted to kill themselves, but some had had a change of heart on that score by the time they were interviewed for this study. The patients often seemed to have additional motives for the acts, such as the desire to hurt people who had angered or rejected them. But it was difficult to assess the degree of importance of such feelings as determinants of suicidal behavior; and even a patient who was quite gravely ill, with a genuine intent to die, could have his suicide attempt precipitated by conflict with his parent or friend. The fact that an apparently trivial circumstance might have triggered a teenager's suicidal act, and that anger might have been mixed with his feelings of hopelessness, in no way indicated that his illness was mild or that he had not actually wanted to die. Nor was a touch of drama necessarily indicative of lack of seriousness. The following note, intended as an obituary for a school newspaper, was written by a 16-year-old white boy with depressive illness who was by all evidence quite earnest in his wish to die:

> "J______ R______ B______, Obituary of:
> J______ R______ B______; born October 17, 1949, died April 8, 1966, American student, educator, fighter, and atheist. Son of department store manager and part-time saleslady. Active participant in high school athletics and extra-curricular school activities. One-time drinker and all-time louse. Heartbreaker and heartbroken, financially insecure and a squanderer. Full-time self-made philosopher who devoted his last days regretting himself and those who knew him. Hated himself more than any other person possibly could have and had misgivings about only one thing he had done. Cause of Death: By his own hand and mind—unforgiven."

In only four of the 45 suicidal patients did the attempts seem patently manipulative, carried out in the presence of observers whose behavior the patients apparently wanted to influence. All four patients were girls who did not fit into a definite diagnostic category.

Medical Seriousness of Attempts

Four of the 45 adolescent suicide attempters had made medically serious attempts. Three of these were unconscious from overdoses of medication, and the fourth patient suffered from exposure to the elements, hunger, and dehydration after lying in a cold barn for 60 hours. Three additional patients were drowsy or semi-conscious from overdoses. The remaining 38 patients had no apparent medical ill-effects from their self-destructive behavior. There was no correlation between psychiatric diagnosis and the medical seriousness of the attempt. Two of the four in the serious group had depressive illness, but two (one of whom had antisocial personality) had disorders principally characterized by behavioral problems. By the same token, one of the sickest patients in the study, a 17-year-old schizophrenic girl with a bizarre premorbid personality, had made three medical unimpressive attempts, once by superficial wrist cuts and twice by small doses of pills. In this sample of patients, one could not use the degree of medical seriousness of a suicide attempt as a guide to the degree of psychiatric impairment, prognosis, or psychologic seriousness of the attempt. A medically trivial attempt was not reassuring.

SUMMARY

Suicide Communication and Attempts

Communication of suicidal intent, by word or action, occurred in two-thirds of the 60 adolescent psychiatric inpatients who were systematically questioned about this. An identical proportion of adult psychiatric inpatients from an earlier study at this hospital[10] had also made such communications. The communications tended to be recent, repetitive, and they were associated with episodes of psychiatric disorder. They were considered serious expressions of distress or desires for death, only rarely as manipulative taunts. Close relatives were by far the most common recipients of communications. Among both teenagers and adults there were six common means of communication: actual suicide attempts, statements by the patient that he wanted to die, that he would be better off dead, that his family would be better off, that he intended to kill himself, and reference to methods of committing suicide. For practical purposes, specific questioning about those items should identify almost all serious communicators in a sample. Among the psychiatrically hospitalized adolescents, suicide communications in general were common features of psychiatric illness and their incidence was not significantly influenced by sex or diagnosis.

Adolescent and adult psychiatric patients were similar with respect to the frequency, methods, and circumstances of suicide communication; however, a significantly higher proportion of teenagers than adults in the comparison sample had actually attempted suicide, despite the fact that the latter group had been sick much longer. This was not unexpected, since evidence from other studies has shown that people who are psychiatrically ill in their teens (which included few of the adult comparison sample) are at greater risk for suicide attempts than are psychiatrically ill adults. In addition, there are indications that there has been an increase in the incidence of adolescent suicide attempts in recent years in this country.[8, 12]

Among the adolescent controls, hospitalized for medical or surgical treatment, suicidal communication only occurred in those who had psychiatric disorders and was significantly more common among patients with prolonged and severe medical illnesses.

Actual suicide attempts had occurred in 44 (40%) of the 110 teenage psychiatric inpatients and in only one control. These were usually drug ingestion, and only four attempts were medically serious. Attempts were significantly more frequent among girls, among typical depressives of either sex, and among the more seriously ill patients of either sex (if the serious illness was dominated by depressive affect). Suicidal behavior was absent in mania, and rare among the schizophrenic and schizoaffective patients.

Suicide attempts were more often a feature of psychiatric disorders in the later than in the earlier teenage years. When attempts did occur before the age of 16, the attempters were almost invariably girls who were "undiagnosed," their illness not fulfulling the criteria for an established psychiatric syndrome in this study. Attempts among boys were associated with the typical depressive syndrome in half the cases, whereas more girl attempters had behavioral problems, for example, traits of hysteria and antisocial personality, along with their depressive affect.

Among the adolescents, neither suicide communications in general, nor suicide attempts in particular, were associated with social class, religion, type or amount of sexual experience, bereavement, alcohol or drug abuse, duration of psychiatric illness, or family history of suicide. But girls who tried to kill themselves had a significantly higher proportion of sick parents, especially fathers with alcoholism.

Psychiatric disorder was a necessary precondition for a suicide attempt, but when viewed in the total context of a patient's illness, such an act was a rare event, usually occurring only once or twice even in an illness of long duration. It seldom seemed of predominant importance compared to other features of the illness. One-third of the suicide attempters had made their attempts without having any psychiatric care-seeking associated with the events and without telling anyone about them until much later.

The fact that an apparently trivial circumstance might have triggered a sick teenager's suicidal act, and that feelings of anger might have been mixed with his feelings of hopelessness, in no way indicated that his illness was mild or that he did not actually intend to die. Similarly, one could not use the degree of medical seriousness of a suicide attempt as a guide to the degree of psychiatric impairment, prognosis, or psychologic seriousness of the attempt. A medically trivial attempt was not reassuring.

Suicidal communications and attempts were symptoms of psychiatric illnesses and did not occur in their absence. They were not features of "adolescence" or "immaturity."

REFERENCES

1. Murphy, G. E., and Robins, E. Social factors in suicide. JAMA *199:* 303–308, 1967.
2. Robins, E., Murphy, G. E., Wilkinson, R. J., Jr., Gassner, S., and Kayes, J. Some clinical considerations in the prevention of suicide based on a study of 134 successful suicides. Am. J. Public Health. *49:* 888–899, 1959.
3. Schmidt, E., O'Neal, P., and Robins, E. Evaluation of suicide attempts as guide to therapy: clinical and follow-up study of 109 patients. J.A.M.A., *155:* 549–557, 1954.
4. Stengel, E., and Cook, N. G. *Attempted Suicide: Its Social Significance and Effects.* Maudsley Monograph No. 4. London, Chapman and Hall, 1958.
5. Robins, E., Gassner, S., Kayes, J., Wilkinson, R. H., Jr., and Murphy, G. E. The communication of suicidal intent: a study of 134 consecutive cases of successful (completed) suicides. Am. J. Psychiatry *115:* 724–733, 1959.
6. Dorpat, T. L., and Ripley, H. S. A study of suicide in the Seattle area. Compr. Psychiatry *1:* 349–359, 1960.
7. Ettinger, R. W. Suicides in a group of patients who had previously attempted suicide. Acta Psychiatr. Scand. *40:* 363–378, 1964.
8. Seiden, R. H. *Suicide among Youth.* Supplement to the Bulletin of Suicidology. U.S.P.H.S. Publication No. 1971, 1969.
9. Jacobziner, H. Attempted suicides in adolescents. JAMA *191:* 7–12, 1965.
10. DeLong, W. B., and Robins, E. The communication of suicidal intent prior to psychiatric hospitalization; a study of 87 patients. Am. J. Psychiatry *117:* 695–705, 1961.
11. Morrison, J. R., Hudgens, R. W., and Barchha, R. G. Life events and psychiatric illness. Br. J. Psychiatry *114:* 423–432, 1968.
12. Murphy, G. E. Unpublished (cited by permission).
13. Reiss, A. J., Jr. *Occupations and Social Status.* New York, The Free Press of Glencoe, Inc., 1961.

6

"Psychosis" and the problem of schizophrenia

THE WORD "PSYCHOSIS"

If one takes the matter of psychiatric diagnosis seriously, restricting one's self to the use of terms which designate well established syndromes with characteristic courses over time, "psychosis" is not a useful diagnostic label. However, the term continues in common parlance among physicians, because a word is needed to connote severe mental illness and "psychotic" is less pejorative than "mad." The American Psychiatric Association's *Diagnostic and Statistical Manual of Mental Disorders* (DSM II, 1968)[1] acknowledges that it is usually the severity of a disorder which leads to its designation as a psychosis: "... Mental functioning is sufficiently impaired to interfere grossly with ... capacity to meet the ordinary demands of life." Thus the term can be used to cover a varied range of illnesses, both those which are characterized by demonstrable organic brain damage and those which are not. This imprecision is further compounded because in DSM II the word is also applied to patients who may not at the moment be very sick, but who have an illness (*e.g.*, mild depression or hypomania) which, if they suffered from a severe form of it, would render them incapable of rational thinking and behavior, that is, "psychotic" in the usual sense.

For these reasons it might be well if the word, psychosis, were dropped from our official diagnostic nomenclature and only used as a polite synonym for madness. We have followed that practice in this book.

CONFUSION OF "PSYCHOSIS" WITH "SCHIZOPHRENIA"

The foregoing considerations are relevant to the subject of schizophrenia in adolescents. Many psychiatrists, especially in the United States, have applied the diagnosis of schizophrenia in uncritical fashion to all teenagers with severe mental disorders, whatever the form and course of the illnesses, and to many who were merely eccentric, for example, socially withdrawn or unpredictable. This practice may, in the first place, result from a disposition by some psychiatrists not to take the process of diagnosis very seriously. Second, since schizophrenia as originally described by

Kraepelin[2] customarily begins in youth, there may be a tendency to give this label to some patients simply on the basis of an early age of onset. Third, many psychiatrists view depression and mania simply as extreme moods rather than illnesses, and believe that these moods are usually reactions to events. Therefore, when a depressed or manic teenager talks or acts in an irrational manner which, moreover, makes no sense in terms of prior events, there is a tendency to call him schizophrenic, even though affective symptoms dominate the clinical picture.

The result of all this in some quarters has been to broaden the diagnostic criteria for schizophrenia to a point that the term becomes useless either in describing a clinical picture or predicting outcome. In the current study, however, we have restricted ourselves to a narrower definition of schizophrenia, using the following criteria:

1. An impairing psychiatric illness which is a change from previous state, which cannot be accounted for on the basis of organic brain disease, and in which symptoms or disability have persisted since onset, although the longitudinal course may be characterized by great changes in the severity of the disability.
2. A persistent disorder of the form of thought (*e.g.*, concept formation, comprehension, or association), or at least two of the following: perceptual disturbance (for example, hallucinations), thought content disturbance, and ideas of passivity.
3. Blunted or incongruous affect.
4. Bizarre or withdrawn behavior.
5. No other diagnosis likely.

DISTINCTION BETWEEN "SCHIZOPHRENIA" AND "UNDIAGNOSED, SCHIZOAFFECTIVE"

It will be noted that we did not diagnose schizophrenia if there was evidence of complete recovery at any time since onset. Our criteria were also stringent in that they required disturbance in three areas—thought, affect, and behavior. And they required that the disorder be impairing: mere eccentricity was not considered to be schizophrenia. These criteria follow the general guidelines of Kraepelin's description of the syndrome. They also take into account the finding of previous workers (for example, Eitinger, *et al.*[3] Welner and Strömgren,[4] Vaillant[5]) that acute affect-laden, remitting states, which may resemble schizophrenia at some point, may be essentially different from "nuclear" or "process" schizophrenia. In fact, such states often resemble manic-depressive illness in their benign outcome, response to ECT, high incidence of affective illness among patients' relatives, and later occurrence of depression in some patients themselves. For these reasons, some workers have suggested that these states may at times be atypical variants of bipolar affective illness (see Clayton, *et al.*[6]). Nevertheless, since the cross-sectional clinical picture of such conditions often resembles schizophrenia, and since they are customarily so classified, they are considered in the current chapter and called "undiagnosed, schizoaffective."

CLINICAL HETEROGENEITY WITHIN THE GROUP DIAGNOSED AS SCHIZOPHRENIC

Even when one restricts himself to the above stringent criteria for making a diagnosis of schizophrenia, he must acknowledge that patients who fit this description are a very mixed group. For example, a patient with onset in his early teens who deteriorates into permanent silliness, muteness, and bizarre posturing is very different from one who develops chronic hallucinations and delusions of reference in his late 20's but maintains an intact personality and continues to work and to function socially. Thus two patients bearing the same diagnosis may have two separate disorders which differ from each other in some essential way, as yet undetermined.

The varieties of clinical pictures seen in schizophrenia have led writers to develop various systems of subclassification which are as much in dispute today as they were 80 years ago. It is sobering to read the early descriptions by Kraepelin and Bleuler and their attempts at classification and to realize that medical science has not progressed very far in its understanding of this disorder (or these disorders) during the past three-quarters of a century. This is despite the fact that many longitudinal studies have been done during that time and that systematic investigations into brain pathology began over 50 years ago.

STUDIES OF CAUSE

Still, hope lies in the direction of further clinical and family studies and in the refinements of techniques of investigation in biochemistry, physiology, ultrastructural pathology, and so forth. Theories of the "essential" nature of the schizophrenic syndrome abound, but doubt has been cast on much of the work when independent investigators have failed to replicate the findings of previous workers or when researchers have failed to use clinically homogeneous groups as their study populations. So far there has been no convincing explanation of the nature and cause of schizophrenia, either by those who study the syndrome in the laboratory or those who study family interaction.

The studies of Kallman,[7] Slater,[8] Heston,[9] and others over the years point to an inherited basis for the illness in many schizophrenics. But no one knows exactly what is inherited, what makes the illness become clinically apparent in a susceptible individual, or what factors—inherited, intrauterine, or environmental—are responsible for the discordance for the illness observed in some identical twins. Moreover, other careful work by Slater *et al.*[10] has demonstrated that epilepsy, after a course of 10 or 20 years, may evolve into an illness that resembles chronic schizophrenia in all respects, despite the absence of familial predisposition. This suggests that there may be more than one neuropathological process leading to a particular clinical picture.

Psychiatry's state of ignorance about schizophrenia has persisted for many decades, and is a measure of how very far we have yet to go as a scientific discipline, despite our ability to alleviate schizophrenic symptoms by some measures, such as the administration of phenothiazines.

This chapter, presenting the clinical and social pictures of schizophrenia and "schizoaffective" illness in 14 adolescents is an examination of the background, course, and consequences of these disorders in a youthful population. The purpose of this presentation is to add clarity to the classification of mental disorders among adolescents by the use of strict diagnostic criteria and to form the basis for a follow-up of these same patients into adulthood.

SCHIZOPHRENIC ADOLESCENTS IN THIS STUDY

General Considerations

Six psychiatric inpatients (and no controls) met our diagnostic criteria for schizophrenia, and a seventh was "undiagnosed, most like schizophrenia." The last was a boy with a chronic illness of insidious onset who did not have quite enough symptoms to qualify for the research diagnosis. These seven adolescents will be considered together as schizophrenics. They fit the clinical picture of early process or nuclear schizophrenia, but socially they did not fit the stereotype of such patients. For example, because they were still quite young, most had not yet deteriorated to a great degree, and they were not of below average intelligence or lower socioeconomic status. On the contrary, most were bright. The average I.Q. was 110, the range 77 to 147, with only two of the seven patients below 108, and they were from the middle or upper social classes. On the Duncan socioeconomic index their mean was 56, compared to a mean of 48 for all 110 psychiatric inpatients. Only two patients came from families below the white collar level, and in no case was the family wage earner unemployed or unskilled. Such schizophrenics may be fairly representative of the middle class American adolescents with this illness found in private psychiatric hospitals.

Family Backgrounds

As mentioned, the families of the schizophrenics were of the middle social class or higher. In addition, there was a low incidence of family psychopathology or disruption. Five of the seven patients were living with both natural parents. One of their five fathers had been a heavy drinker (not enough to qualify for the diagnosis, alcoholism) and one mother had been hospitalized for a "nervous breakdown" at about age 30 and had recovered.

The other two patients were the only schizophrenics who came from disrupted homes. In one of these cases, the mother had divorced an alcoholic father, who was subsequently killed in an automobile accident. There had been two suicides on the mother's side of that family. In the other case, the patient lived in an orphanage in Ireland for the first three and one-half years of his life, then he was adopted and raised in America. Nothing was known of his natural family.

Predominantly negative feelings on the part of the patients toward their parents were unusual, being expressed toward only three of the 14 functional parents. This was in contrast to the greater prevalence of such negative attitudes among the psychiatric inpatients with some other disorders.

The seven schizophrenic subjects had a total of 14 siblings, none of whom had psychiatric illness. And although there were a few psychiatrically ill remote relatives, none apparently was schizophrenic. Depression and alcoholism were the only identifiable disorders among them.

Premorbid Scholastic and Social Adjustment

The generally above-average intelligence of the patients has already been mentioned. All but one entered school at the appropriate age, and only two patients were held back academically, both of them in first grade. As nearly as we could determine, the onset of schizophrenia in these seven adolescents occurred at a mean age of 13.3 years (range 12 to 17). Academic and social performance was thereafter impaired, of course. Three patients had dropped out of school by the time of the study (mean age 16.3 years), and peer relationships were disturbed. Three patients had never dated, whereas four had done so, but not frequently. Only one patient had had heterosexual intercourse, and two had had homosexual experience, although this was not extensive. It is striking that there was no socially delinquent activity among the seven schizophrenic adolescents, either before or during their illnesses: no history of truancy, fights, disciplinary suspensions from school, or arrests. Only two of the group drank (a minimal amount of alcohol) and none had abused alcohol or used illegal drugs.

Premorbid Brain Damage

There was definite evidence of premorbid insult to the central nervous system in three of the seven patients, including the two who came from disrupted homes:

Y-009 had onset at age 17 and was 19 at the time of our study. At age five he had had measles complicated by encephalitis with coma and convulsions. He was notably "nervous" and tremulous from age five to 12, was quiet and serious and never made close friends. This was the patient who had the alcoholic father, later killed, and two suicides in his mother's family.

Y-035 had onset at age 12 and was 17 at the time of admission. She had had febrile convulsions at age two, fractured her skull at age seven, and had headaches for a year thereafter.

Y-039, 12 years old at onset and 17 at the time of our study, was in an orphanage until age three and one-half years, then adopted. He had a skull fracture at age six, then was hyperactive and underachieved in school. He never fit in socially, and was the butt of jokes in his peer group.

Two of the remaining four patients may have had brain injury. One, with a normal premorbid personality, began to have the insidious onset of schizophrenia after an automobile accident and "whiplash" injury. The other, although without a prior history of head trauma or CNS disorder, had a markedly assymetrical skull on radiographic examination at the time of her study admission.

The Clinical Picture of Schizophrenia

Premorbid Symptoms

In an illness of insidious onset it is not possible to date with certainty the month, or sometimes even the year, in which it began. For this reason, it was often impossible to distinguish premorbid traits in our schizophrenics (such as eccentricity, withdrawal, and affective disturbances) from symptoms of the illness itself. Examination of our material suggests that such distinctions may be artificial in many cases and that so-called premorbid personality traits in schizophrenia may simply be early symptoms, occurring even in childhood, of an illness which is seldom fully expressed until adolescence.

Recognizing this problem, we nevertheless assigned ages of onset for our schizophrenic subjects, scoring the beginning of the illness as the appearance of multiple symptoms and of social or scholastic disability. At the time of admission, two patients were 13 years old, three were 17, one was 18 and one 19 (mean 16.3 years). Onset had been at age 12 for three patients, at 13 for two, 14 for one, and 17 for one (mean 13.3 years). The patient whose onset was age 14 had had no remarkable premorbid traits, but the patient whose onset was 17 had been nervous, tremulous, isolated, and unaffectionate since at least age five. So only one of the seven schizophrenics had failed to show definite peculiarity by age 13.

Three of the seven patients were described as having symptoms or abnormal personality traits *prior* to the age of onset. These were the same three patients who had had insults to the central nervous system (discussed in the previous section). The premorbid features included nervousness, tremors, social isolation, and unaffectionate nature (patient Y-009); introversion, suicidal and homicidal ideation, and obsessions (Y-035); hyperactivity, scholastic underachievement, social withdrawal, and "oddness" (Y-039). All these symptoms later appeared as significant features of the patients' full-blown illnesses. One might speculate that the CNS disorders were in part causative factors in the schizophrenic illnesses of these patients, or perhaps that brain damage contributed to the development in childhood of some schizophrenic symptoms by patients who were destined to develop the full syndrome in their teens anyway.

Onset

The mode of onset varied, as shown in the descriptions below; but affective symptoms, especially depressive moods, were very prominent early in most patients' illnesses. This was despite the fact that the clinical pictures were eventually not dominanted by depression, and that these patients were schizophrenic by strict criteria.

> Y-009—This white boy had been quiet, serious, socially isolated, and nervous since having measles encephalitis at age five. The illness seemed to begin insidiously at age 17, early in his senior year of high school, with decreased talking to his parents, loss of his sense of humor, irritability, and unwillingness to do household chores. Initially, these seemed accentuations of his premorbid personality traits. He become preoccupied with the fact that his old athletic coach had left and that the new one seemed less interested in him. He began to complain of a chronically painful ankle, although no damage was found on examination. His grades in that final year of high school dropped, but with tutoring he graduated. During the following summer, he announced his desire to go to California, but he became panicky after a few days there, and his father had to go get him. During the succeeding few months he became increasingly bewildered, sometimes becoming lost while driving. He entered college in the fall, but "gave up" and left in the first semester. Back home, he began to shut himself in his room and to hide in the basement when friends came to visit. He showed no depression,

seemed in a daze, but said that nothing was wrong with him. It was about 15 months from probable onset to the full development of the illness.

Y-031—This was a black girl who had no history of psychiatric symptoms prior to the onset of her illness at age 13. Then she rather abruptly began to believe that men passing by her in cars were imitating her to make fun of her. About a month later, she began hearing the voices of young men calling her and saying good things about other girls. The voices were clearly heard and seemed to come from far away. She became moody, believed herself to be too thin, and began to eat a great deal. The thought that the men in the passing cars were also bothering her family caused her to think of suicide and to look for a knife, but she made no attempt nor did she appear afraid. All this went on for two months before she told anyone it was happening.

Y-035—This white girl with a childhood history of febrile seizures, skull fracture and headaches, was not noticeably ill, as far as her parents were concerned, until she was 16. However, the patient herself convincingly gave a history of chronic unhappiness and death wishes since age 12 with suicidal wrist slashes at that time and a year later. She said that when she was 14 she began to think of killing her father and brothers by poison, but did not try it because she was afraid of getting caught. From her early teens she also had some handwashing and counting compulsions. When she was 16, she gradually developed the delusion that there was a conspiracy at school and that one particular boy was following her. She told no one of this when it began. Her illness finally became obvious to her parents later that same year when they found her walking beside a highway in the rain at a time she was supposed to be in school. She had a blank facial expression, rigid extremities, and the information she volunteered made no sense. Only then was she taken to a doctor.

Y-039 ("Undiagnosed, most like schizophrenia")—This was a white boy adopted from an orphanage at three and one-half years of age. He was hyperactive in elementary school, played with objects instead of studying, and talked to himself. He described himself as always having been unhappy, but his mother said he was "happy-go-lucky." As a child he was overweight and odd. He was always teased for this and for dwelling on subjects of warfare in his conversation and annoying others. At about age 12, he began acting out elaborate fantasies concerning the American Civil War, using toy soldiers, and going to the nearby cemetery where General Sherman is buried to reenact battles. He would also have episodes lasting ten or 15 minutes, usually when awake in bed, in which he would believe himself to be "in" the Civil War or the television program, "Gunsmoke." At some time between age 12 and 15 he began hearing his thoughts and voices criticizing him, which continued. Also, irrelevant ideas would suddenly come into his consciousness and interfere with his schoolwork. All these phenomena continued and intensified over a five-year period.

At age 16, five months before admission, he began to have suicidal thoughts, irritability, and insomnia. He became more socially isolated. This culminated, shortly before admission, in his jumping from the roof of his house in a suicide attempt after schoolmates had been picking on him. (It is interesting to note the long duration of psychopathology in this boy before his first referral for care.)

Y-045—This black girl was well until age 14. She then was in an automobile accident in which she received a "whiplash" injury and had a stiff neck for a week thereafter. During the subsequent few weeks, there was insidious development of stiffness in her whole body. Psychiatric symptoms developed gradually over a period of six months after the injury. She began losing interest in school, became worried about sex instruction, and could not remember things. She became tense and wept frequently. About four months after the accident, she thought someone she knew was passing by in a car several times a day. She began to hear voices, see visions, and imagine that people were talking about her. She felt guilty and wanted to die.

At the time of onset her illness resembled depression more than schizophrenia. But over the next three years before the study admission the course became typical of schizophrenia. By that time she was 17 years old.

Y-052—This black girl also developed affective symptoms at the onset of what later turned out to be typical and unremitting schizophrenia. She had been happy and had friends, although she had a low I.Q. (77) and did marginal work in school. At the beginning of the school year, when she was 12 years old, she was placed in a special class. She disliked this, cried, and over the next three months became "sleepy-eyed" and very quiet. During this period of onset she began to walk around the house at two to three a.m., then began to talk to herself, whether alone or with other people. She began to hear voices telling her to jump out the window. She cried a great deal, but had no feelings of guilt or self-depreciation. After three months, these symptoms intensified to the point that hospitalization was required. (The admission during which she entered our study was one year later, and her course had by then become typically schizophrenic.)

Y-058—The brightest (I.Q. 146) of the schizophrenics was this white boy who had a long period of illness, from age 13 to 18, before his family realized that something was wrong. In his case as in others' depression played a role in the presenting clinical picture. The patient, who appeared a reliable historian, reported that when he was 13 he realized he had been involved in elaborate fantasies for as long as he could remember. At that age he gradually came to believe in their reality, thought himself to be the leader and descendent of a lost race which had once been on earth, then departed through space to the star Procyon. A voice, called "Orion," told him that his mission was to bring this race to power by unspecified means. As he grew older he heard other voices, including his own thoughts, and the voices began using vile language when he was 15. At that age he began to be depressed and worried. He then developed an irrational hatred for one of his teachers, which led to his attacking the teacher with a pen-knife after slight provocation. He was expelled from that school.

During the succeeding three years he developed hypochrondriacal preoccupation, and gradually had more prominent depressive symptoms. By age 17, he was having death wishes, heading his automobile toward trees on several occasions, but losing his nerve and swerving back onto the road. Despite all this he graduated from high school and entered college. Other symptoms soon developed: he would get words mixed up, feel that he was someone else, be easily tired, have delusions that he was spied upon, that his thoughts were being read, that his car was wired for bombing, and that an alien voice at times took over his body. At other times he would develop the sensation that his body was nothing, and he was then unable to see or hear for a few minutes. He developed severe headaches and back pain. Finally, he began to have delusions that one of his college teachers was against him, according to information from his voices. This symptom led him to seek psychiatric help on his own, because he had partial insight into the illogical nature of his delusions.

Beginning almost a year before his coming to psychiatric care, he kept a diary, which detailed his bewilderment and fear and which provides a good example of the schizophrenic thought content of a very bright and articulate youth. Excerpts from this diary follow: Dec. 1, 1966. "They are trying to destroy me by thought-suggestion. I have been fighting it but I am growing weaker and they are growing stronger. They, like me, are not of this earth. Or am I from earth? It dates back to Nov. 13, 1964. I am confused. They cannot harm me physically, but they can take control of my brain and make me do their wishes. They have taken control of me for several seconds, but then have lost control. This is not good. I am fighting a losing battle. Can Mr. ____ be connected with them? I doubt the possibility. I fear that I can't last much longer. No one can help me. I know they wouldn't believe me. I must fight this by myself. If you have noticed me depressed, now you understand. This not a psychosis or neurosis, or any other mental disease. It is all returning: the preparations, the long struggle, the battle, the fear, the boy, the warp, and the escape." ... Jan. 19, 1967. "Again have foiled their attempts on my life. Paranoia prominent. Manic-depressive state prevails. Sean (as I call him) does exist and is one of them. Mrs. ____ may understand. Or think I was completely mad. (Friday night, they got J____. They obtained no information but produced temporary amnesia.) Sense of time fading. Sense of responsibility almost gone. Brain deteriorating. Hard to concentrate. Consciousness drifts into subconsciousness. Awareness eroding. Tension increasing." ... Jan. 30, 1967. "Motor movements deteriorating. They want me back. All previous memories returning. They have won." ... Jan. 31, 1967. "C____ died last night at 7:10 p.m. May he rest in peace. Am being forced to see doctor. What will he find? I think it is mono." ... Feb. 23, 1967. "I must be going mad. Sleep comes hard these days. It is terrifying. They are everywhere. Last night I took 15 aspirins. But I might be saved. Tuesday was a bitch." ... Mar. 6, 1967. "Am feeling very weird. Superior force may be present." ... "I love N____, but I broke her heart because of my irrational actions. Even talking and thinking are hard, at times, impossible."

Fully Developed Clinical Picture

Much of the clinical picture among our schizophrenic teenagers is detailed in the above section about onset. Even when depression was a prominent early symptom, it had become less impressive compared to other symptoms by the time of the study admission. By that time the adolescents appeared quite strange, and their affect was incongruous. The symptoms of the fully developed syndrome are listed in Table 31. In

TABLE 31
Current Symptoms Reported for Seven Schizophrenics

Symptom	Number of Patients with Symptom
Auditory hallucinations	At least 6
Depressed or sad	At least 5
Thoughts of suicide	At least 5
Decreased interest	At least 4
School or work disability	At least 4
Trouble thinking	At least 4
People reading mind	At least 4
Hopelessly sick or mixed-up	At least 4
Guilty or worthless	At least 4
Nausea or vomiting	At least 3
Insomnia	At least 3
Temper, rages, or fighting	At least 3
Suicide attempt	At least 2
People watching you	At least 2
People following you	At least 2
People plotting for or against you	At least 2
Things seem changed	At least 2
Visual hallucinations	At least 2

comparison with the other patients in the study the schizophrenics were less communicative and gave fewer positive responses. We suspected that there were many false negative answers to questions in our symptom checklist, and one of the seven patients gave such a sparse history that his story had to be pieced together from reports of earlier hospitalizations and from the interview with his parents. Thus the symptom list in Table 30 is affected by under-reporting of psychopathology. Affective symptoms were reported frequently, because they occurred in almost every case, but they did not ultimately dominate the clinical picture. Several symptoms which were frequent in other disorders were rarely reported by the schizophrenics. For example, nervousness, headache, weight loss, fatigue, and fast thoughts were each reported by only one patient.

A symptom checklist can not give the flavor of an illness. This can best be conveyed by describing the clinical picture while our patients were at their worst.

> Y-009—Prior to the study admission this 19-year-old boy stayed in his room, preoccupied, refusing to see family or friends, not changing his clothes. He would stare at a book in his lap or at the clothes his mother would put out for him to wear. On the way to the hospital, he was verbally abusive to the ambulance attendant and was tied to the litter.

Upon entering the hospital he was unkempt, turned his face away from the interviewer, and gave brief, stereotyped, unreliable answers to questions after prolonged delays. He was uncooperative.

Y-031—This 13-year-old girl had an increase in the "voices" which she had been hearing, and became convinced that her psychiatrist, parents, and the people whose voices she heard were in league against her. Upon admission she appeared neatly dressed. Her manner was calm and quiet throughout the interview and her mood unremarkable. Her sensorium was clear. She believed in her delusions, but concluded that the way she could help herself was to study harder in school.

Y-035—This 17-year-old girl became increasingly fearful prior to admission, with homicidal and suicidal ideation. She persisted in her belief that there was a conspiracy against her and that she was being followed. "I'll kill myself rather than let them kill me." She could hear footsteps outside her room, and heard a buzzing in her head whenever she thought of killing her family or herself. She had the visual illusion of a space around objects, like the "ghost image" on television. She became fearful of riding in automobiles and afraid that buildings might catch fire.

Upon admission she was matter-of-fact, with bland, cold affect when talking of her desire to kill her family. She seemed baffled by any question requiring elaboration of prior statements, but she was oriented and easily answered questions to which a yes-or-no response was sufficient. She believed in her delusions and did not believe herself to be psychiatrically ill.

Y-039 ("Undiagnosed, most like schizophrenia")—This 17-year-old boy had increasing feelings of sadness and irritability, along with suicidal thoughts in the few weeks prior to admission. His audible thoughts continued, and he began hearing voices of other people criticizing him. He continued his preoccupation with the American Civil War, acting out elaborate fantasies of battles. Upon admission, he was polite and cooperative, seeming not at all depressed. He became animated, eager, and intense whenever he spoke of the Civil War, with his fists clinched and a grimacing face. There was no push of speech or tangentiality. He was oriented. He remained without apparent depression during his hospital stay, but annoyed other patients with his constant talk of war. He was accused by another patient of making a homosexual advance toward him.

Y-045—This 17-year-old girl experienced increasing auditory hallucinations and delusions of reference prior to the study admission. She would become agitated and fearful, rushing at people at times. She became poorly groomed, ate excessively, and gained weight.

Upon admission she appeared about 12 years old rather than 17. She was short and obese. Her movements were slow. Her flow of speech was at times normal, at other times halting. Sentences would trail off into mumbling. Her mood was unremarkable. She was oriented to time, place, and person, but was unable to give a chronologic account of events. Her speech was tangiential. She believed that anyone who was with her controlled her actions. She heard voices, felt a snake on her face. She believed that she had been pregnant ever since she was eight years old, and that she had drowned at age eight. She spoke incomprehensibly, with some neologisms. She had "a grauma, a dying on the cross." "This thing eats everything I eat, doesn't let me have any food." "Grout. That is what the nurses said to say: and goshes and gender and grauma."

Y-052—This 13-year-old girl remained out of school following a prior psychiatric hospitalization 10 months before the study admission. She was withdrawn, had crying spells, heard voices, and talked to herself. Her affect was flat and inappropriate, and she had a short attention span. The study hospital admission was precipitated by her suddenly beginning to scream, run around the house, and attempt to jump out the window.

Upon examination she assumed awkward postures, grimaced, and laughed inappropriately at times. She was periodically sullen and uncooperative. Her speech was frequently blocked, with long latency of response, and at times an absence of response. Finally, she stopped answering questions in the research interview and began moving her lips as if talking to herself. Her mood was neither elated nor depressed. She could not give a chronologic account of her history and was disoriented to time.

Y-058—The clinical course leading to hospitalization of this 18-year-old boy was described in the above section of this chapter. Upon admission he was polite, sincere, and not at all guarded. However, he was tense and smoked constantly. His mood was appropriate and unremarkable. At one point in the interview he suddenly appeared preoccupied, his eyes narrowed, and he looked at the interviewer suspiciously. Upon questioning he admitted to hearing voices at that moment. He believed in his mission to lead a lost race back to earth from a distant planet.

Course and Outcome

At the time of this study, the seven schizophrenic patients had a mean age of 16.3 (range 13 to 19) and had been sick a mean of 3.0 years (range six months to five years). As indicated in the case histories, the onset and course of their disorders were variable from patient to patient, and symptoms present for months or years might have escaped the notice of patients' parents and persisted without the patients themselves commenting upon them. These adolescents generally either lacked insight into the fact that they were sick at all, or lacked insight into the way in which they were sick. For example, patient Y-052 identified his problem as "depression," not his elaborately systematized delusions, and Y-009, who was very withdrawn, said he came in "because I had a difference of opinion with my parents." Both these statements were correct, as far as they went, but in each case the patient was unaware that his most striking symptoms were pathologic.

Despite the prolonged course of their illnesses, the patients had experienced relatively little prior hospitalization. Three of the seven had never been admitted before, three had one prior admission, and one patient had two admissions. Cumulative prior time in hospitals was more than three months for only two patients.

During hospitalization at Renard, five of the seven patients improved. All but one received phenothiazines, and two of these also received tricyclic antidepressants. Three patients received electrotherapy, one of them having 30 treatments with no clinical improvement. Length of index hospitalization ranged from nine to 138 days, with a median of 19 days and a mean of 40 days.

In general, little comfort could be derived from the improvement during hospitalization reported for five of the seven patients. Based upon their clinical course up to the time of the study, chronic symptoms and long-term phenothiazine use seemed in prospect for most of these young people.

THE "UNDIAGNOSED, SCHIZOAFFECTIVE" ADOLESCENTS

General Considerations

There were seven patients who had acute, affect-laden illnesses in which features of both schizophrenia and manic-depressive illness were so prominent that we could not exclude either diagnosis. As mentioned earlier, there is controversy as to the proper classification of such patients, with support cited for the views that they are schizophrenics, or atypical manic-depressives, or victims of a third type illness. Based upon our clinical experience and from evidence cited in the literature, it is safe to predict that some of these patients will be found at follow-up to be typically schizophrenic (with affective features becoming progressively less prominent), that others will have had typical manic or depressive episodes, and thus have established themselves as having bipolar affective disorder, and that still others will remain unclassifiable.

Seven subjects received the schizoaffective label. Five were girls, two boys; five were white, two black. Their ages ranged from 14 to 19 (mean 16.71 years). The average age of onset of the first episode was 16.57 years, much older than for the schizophrenics (13.3 years), and comparable to those patients with bipolar affective disorder whose first episode had been mania (16.3 years).

Family Backgrounds

Five of the seven schizoaffectives lived with their natural parents, whereas the homes of the other two had been disrupted by divorce when the patients were one year old and 12 years old, respectively. The families of origin were of a social class comparable to our total subject population (mean Duncan S.E.I. 49.3), and lower than the families of the seven schizophrenic subjects. Only one family wage earner was in the professional class, two were in crafts or skilled trades, one semi-skilled, two unskilled, one unemployed.

Six of the 14 parents had a history of psychiatric illness by our criteria. One mother and two fathers were alcoholic, and one mother and two fathers had had depressive illness. (Two fathers and one mother had been in jail, but no parent had an antisocial personality.) Four of the six ill parents had been hospitalized for their psychiatric disorders. Thus 43% of the parents were ill, a proportion a bit higher than that of the entire psychiatrically ill subject group in our study, and six (86%) of the seven schizoaffective adolescents had at least one ill parent. None of the parents had died, and none of the 26 siblings had died or had a psychiatric illness.

Premorbid Scholastic and Social Adjustment

Among the seven adolescents, there had been no complications at the time of their mothers' pregnancies, and no problems at birth. I.Q.'s for the five who were tested ranged from 82 to 118 (mean 102.8). Only one patient had had academic problems, having been held back one year in elementary school. None of the seven schizoaffectives had a prior history of fights, truancy, expulsion, arrests, or abuse of drugs or alcohol, and all were enrolled in school at the time of the study. All the schizoaffective subjects had dated, although only two began before age 15. One was married, none of the others had been engaged, and only one of the unmarried patients had ever had sexual intercourse. Thus there was an absence of antisocial behavior or predictors of such behavior in the years preceding the onset of the schizoaffective illnesses.

Premorbid Difficulties

The onset of schizoaffective illness was acute and recent in all seven cases, and it was thus possible to get a retrospective description of the premorbid status from the patients and their parents. Only one of the seven teenagers was totally free of premorbid psychiatric difficulty. Of the others, Y-066, a 17-year-old white boy, had been effeminate and homosexual, with few friends. For a year prior to the onset of his illness he had spent time in his room, sitting on his bed making faces at times. He had had occasional temper outbursts. Y-084, a 19-year-old black girl, had not been noticed to be unusual by her parents, but she herself reported having "heard" occasional phrases, perhaps her own thoughts, since age 12, and to have been nervous and self-conscious since age 17, feeling perhaps that people could read her mind. Y-091 was a 15-year-old white girl who had been quiet and shy but not described as abnormally so. From ages eight to 12, she had had nightmares after which she would run to her parents' room, with amnesia for those episodes. At age 14, she hit out occasionally at her parents, and two months before admission she had a low mood for a time after breaking up with a boyfriend. Y-094, a white boy, 14-years-old at onset, had always been shy, lacked motor control in school, and found it difficult to express himself in speaking or writing. Y-099, a 16-year-old white girl, had always been shy and nervous. At age nine, she developed fear of crowds and had fainting spells for a while. When she was 12, she thought someone was plotting against her for a time, and a few months before admission she developed the very brief, inexplicable feeling that her father might kill her mother, because he was talking too loudly. Y-013, although described as having a normal premorbid personality, reported an "overdose" two years before admission. Three of the six patients with premorbid symptoms had a history of head injury with brief unconsciousness, Y-066 at age 13, Y-084 at age 12, Y-094 at age 7. No sequelae were noticed from these injuries, and it was difficult to connect them with either their premorbid difficulties or the stormy onsets of their illnesses, which began much later.

The Clinical Picture of Schizoaffective Illness

The time of onset varied from three days to three months prior to the study admission, with a mean duration of illness of about 35 to 40 days before hospitalization. Only one patient, Y-103, had been ill before. She had developed a schizoaffective picture one year prior to the study admission. That episode had remitted without EST or phenothiazines. All the other patients were in their first episodes at the time of the study.

In contrast to the schizophrenics, the schizoaffectives and their informants reported a plethora of symptoms (Table 32). Marked mood disturbance, hallucinations, and delusions of reference and passivity were invariably present and dominated the clinical picture. Disorientation (to time or place) occurred in only one. Nevertheless, bewilderment and confusion about what was going on was typical. Suicidal thoughts were present in four patients, but suicide had not been the primary concern in seeking admission, either on the part of the patients or their parents. The schizoaffectives were a more clincially uniform group than the schizophrenics. They differed from person to person as to individual thought content, but not as to the form of the illness. All were floridly, dramatically ill, and there was no doubt in their minds or the minds of their families that something was terribly wrong with them. The dominant mood was frantic dysphoria and agony, and the vegetative symptoms and mental content of affective disorder were present in abundance. Three patients were elated at times, and two had grandiose delusions, so that with respect to affect, the schizoaffectives resembled a mixed manic-depressive picture. However,

TABLE 32

Symptoms in Seven Schizoaffective Adolescents

Symptom	
Depression	7
Worry	7
Insomnia	7
People watching you	7
People following you	7
People reading your mind	7
Trouble thinking or concentrating	6
Anorexia	6
Auditory hallucinations	6
Hopelessly sick or mixed-up	5
Decreased interest	5
Not well groomed	5
People plotting for or against you	5
Derealization	5
Things around you are changed	5
Visual hallucinations	5
Death wishes	4
Suicidal thoughts	4
Guilt	4
Trouble with memory	4
Weight loss	4
Receiving messages	4
Self changing	4

the delusions and hallucinations often seemed incongruous with the mood disturbance.

Two case reports are presented here, one of a patient with definite premorbid difficulties, one of a patient with minimal premorbid problems.

Y-066—This white boy (17 years old at the onset of his illness) had temper tantrums at ages two and three, accompanied by head-banging. In his pre-teen years he customarily played with children younger than he. By age 11, he had developed effeminate mannerisms. His schoolmates called him "a queer," and he had few friends. His father would take him hunting, but the boy disliked killing animals. His mother, who was a chronic alcoholic, would beat him at times for no reason. The parents were divorced when he was ten, and he stayed with his father, who later remarried. By his early teens, he had developed occasional episodes, lasting up to several days, of withdrawal and crying. He also continued to have temper tantrums. His first homosexual experience was at age 14, when his brother performed anal intercourse on him. Over the succeeding three years before the onset of his illness he had occasional mutual masturbation with other boys.

The patient's stepmother become increasingly concerned about him by the time he was 16 because of his effeminacy and because he was spending a great deal of time sitting on his bed, making faces. However, at age 17, about two months before the onset of his illness, he became more outgoing, got a part-time job, and went to some parties.

About two weeks before the study admission the patient noticed the onset of depression, with crying spells and death wishes. He developed insomnia, anorexia, nausea, increased sexual urges, and occasional inability to control urination. He thought people were following him and watching him, and that television was sending messages to him and influencing him in ways he could not specify. People could read his mind, and vice-versa. They controlled him by their actions so that when they did something he had to do the same thing, or just the opposite. He felt unreal, confused, and believed he was dead or dying. He would check his pulse to see if his heart was beating. Objects around him seemed changed, as if in a brighter light. He soon developed a feeling of special mission against Communism, ordained by God, whom he saw and talked with. He heard voices, calling him "queer" and other epithets, and he in turn called the voices bad names.

This illness first became obvious to others only four days before admission to Renard Hospital. He became angry and sullen for no apparent reason and confided to his stepmother that someone at school was making remarks about him. Two days before admission he lay his head on his desk at school and would not speak to anyone. At home that night he told his stepmother that he had a plan to outsmart his teachers, classmates, and brother. He could now read minds and had gained power. Whenever he was contradicted he became so angry that his stepmother was terrified, and temporarily took the younger children out of the house. On the day before admission he was confused, could not sit still, and had difficulty answering simple questions. He wore a "blank" facial expression.

Upon admission the patient was disheveled, but cooperative and polite, and spoke in a high-pitched voice. Sometimes he maintained eye contact, at other times he stared into space and said he was listening to voices. He frequently gave answers which appeared unrelated to the questions, then would agree that the answer had been inappropriate and give an appropriate answer. His answers were stereotyped, for example, he would answer "yes, yes" to a question, then correct himself by saying "no, no." In response to questions concerning the chronology and duration of symptoms he characteristically replied "four years" or "two weeks." Frequently he said "my mother is dead, no, my mother is not dead." He also demonstrated motor ambivalence, getting up to get a drink of water, then stopping each time, or when instructed to remove his shoes, taking one off, then putting it back on, then in apparent great impatience, tearing it off again. At times he would shout the answers to questions with great vehemence after he had made ambiguous responses. He described his mood as "nervous." His memory for events of the preceding two weeks was impaired, but he was fully oriented.

Y-103—This white girl was 18 at the time of the study admission, and had had the onset of a remitting illness of a similar type one year before. She first became ill quite abruptly at age 17, when she was noted to give a substandard presentation at school one day. The next evening she abruptly left her boyfriend at a bowling alley and went home, having developed the delusion that a surprise party was being planned for her there. She wandered through the house, calling the name of the boy she had just left. She thought her feet were getting smaller and that her father's suit belonged to her boyfriend. During the next day, she stated that she was going to have a baby who had no father and compared herself to the Virgin Mary. She squirmed and cried out as if she were in labor and asked her mother to deliver the baby. She then developed posturing and occasional muteness, interspersed with talk of fearing death and talk of famous people. She voiced the delusion that President John Kennedy was alive, believed that she was being followed, heard voices, saw visions, and laughed and cried inappropriately. With these symptoms, all of which had developed within 48 hours, she was admitted to another hospital, where she remained for 13 days before her transfer to Renard Hospital, at times mute and stiffly posturing, at other times talking tangentially as if bewildered: "How can someone's hand on yours make you feel better? Did Bobby drown? He was a nice boy, but he didn't go to church much. Did I have an operation? Why do I have a class ring?" After her admission to Renard, she developed a fever and transient sixth nerve palsy. She was transferred to the neurology service where she had an extensive neurologic work-up for suspected encephalitis, with negative results, except for temporarily elevated CSF pressure. Brain biopsy and brain cultures were negative for evidence of encephalitis or any virus infection, as were multiple serologic tests for the known encephalitic viruses. The illness remitted with no specific treatment after a total duration of four months, and was followed by a brief depressive state, in which the patient had no energy or interest, neglected her personal appearance, and talked of death.

She remained entirely well for five to six months. She then developed an episode lasting two weeks of depression, anorexia, decreased interest and energy, inability to concentrate, and thoughts of death and suicide. This remitted, she was well for about two weeks, then gradually developed increased energy, pacing, faster and louder talk, heightened interest in things. She rapidly changed topics for her term paper in school. She reported hearing voices throughout that month. Anorexia, weight loss, and insomnia became increasingly marked, and she was readmitted to Renard Hospital.

Upon admission she had generally flat affect with occasional inappropriate laughter. She admitted that she felt controlled, that she could read minds and was having thoughts put into her head. Voices mocked her. She saw "lights, people, and paper," apparently visual hallucinations. She had the feeling that a snake was crawling over her body and the sensation, perhaps also a haptic hallucination, that she was having sexual intercourse. She was oriented in all respects during the study admission and did not develop fever or neurologic signs during that episode of illness.

Course and Outcome

The periods of hospitalization for schizoaffectives during the study admission ranged from 22 to 63 days, with a mean of 43 and a median of 46 days. This was longer than the stay for manics, depressives, and schizophrenics. Since the patients had acute onset and an affect-laden picture, their psychiatrists anticipated complete recovery, despite the presence of bizarre, schizophrenic-like symptoms. They were treated vigorously: all seven received phenothiazines, and all but one received electrotherapy during the study admission. The exception was Y-103, the patient of a physician who seldom gave that type of treatment.

Five of the seven patients, including the one who did not receive ECT, became completely well and were not readmitted. Two patients, Y-066 and Y-094, the only two boys and the patients with the most persistent premorbid abnormalities, remained ill for at least two years after the study admission and required further hospitalization. They had both been treated vigorously on their first admission and had achieved social remission but retained some symptoms. Repeated hospitalization and vigorous treatment again failed to alleviate their symptoms completely. These two patients appeared destined for a typical schizophrenic course, in contrast to others whose outcome resembled more closely that of affective disorder.

SUMMARY

Schizophrenia and "Undiagnosed, Schizoaffective"

Fourteen psychiatric inpatients are considered in this chapter. Six of them fulfilled our strict criteria for schizophrenia: the patients had never been well since onset; they demonstrated disturbance of thought, behavior, and affect; and no other diagnosis was likely (for example, manic-depressive illness, organic brain syndrome, or drug toxicity). A seventh patient, probably schizophrenic, had too few symptoms to fulfill the criteria, but was considered with the other six. The illnesses of these patients began at a mean age of 13.3 years, and had been present for an average of three years at the time of the study. No patient developed schizophrenia before the age of 12. However, three of the seven patients had a history of insult to the central nervous system in childhood, and these three patients had definite premorbid symptoms which later became distinctive features of their schizophrenic disorders.

Despite the fact that the illnesses of the seven schizophrenics did not resemble any other psychiatric disorder, they were a clinically heterogeneous group, with a variety of types of onset and symptomatology. Depressed mood was a feature early in the course of illness in some patients and was a common precipitant of hospital admission; but depression was not the dominant feature in any of the patients' illnesses. The group had principally three things in common: very early onset (age 13), chronicity, and marked disability. But apart from that, the clinical pictures varied enough from patient to patient to suggest that they may not have all been suffering from the same "essential" disease process, although they all bore the same diagnostic label.

Seven other patients were called schizoaffectives because they had so many features of both schizophrenia and manic-depressive illness that neither syndrome could be excluded from consideration. The schizoaffectives were clinically a much more homogeneous group than the schizophrenics. They had the acute onset of a stormy illness characterized by bewilderment, agonized affect, auditory and visual hallucinations, and delusions of reference and passivity. Five of the seven recovered completely and remained well. They were an average of three years older than the schizophrenics when they first became ill, and some may have had an atypical variety of manic-depressive disorder.

Six patients with schizoaffective illness had premorbid symptoms which were later manifested in the illnesses themselves, although only one had been socially impaired before the abrupt onset of his illness.

The parents of schizoaffectives had a high proportion of incidence of psychiatric illness (43%). This was depression or alcoholism in every case. By contrast, the incidence of illness was low among the parents of schizophrenics (16%), and no relative, primary or remote, was known to have schizophrenia.

There was no history of antisocial behavior, drug abuse, alcohol excess, or school discipline problems among the schizophrenics and schizoaffectives. The patients were generally of middle or higher social class, with at least average intelligence.

REFERENCES

1. *DSM II: Diagnostic and Statistical Manual of Mental Disorders* (second edition). Washington, American Psychiatric Association, 1968.
2. Kraepelin, E. *Dementia Praecox and Paraphrenia* (trans. Barclay, R. M.). Edinburgh, Livingstone, 1919.
3. Eitinger, L., Laane, C. L., and Langfeldt, C. The prognostic value of the clinical picture and the therapeutic value of physical treatment in schizophrenia and the schizophreniform states. Acta Psychiatr. Neurol. Scand. *33:* 33–55, 1958.
4. Welner, J., and Strömgren, E. Clinical and genetic studies on benign schizophreniform psychoses based on a follow-up. Acta Psychiatr. Neurol. Scand. *33:* 377–399, 1958.
5. Vaillant, G. E. Prospective prediction of schizophrenic remission. Arch. Gen. Psychiatry *11:* 509–518, 1964.
6. Clayton, P. J., Rodin, L., and Winokur, G. Family history studies: III. Schizo-

affective disorder, clinical and genetic factors including a one to two year follow-up. Comp. Psychiatry *9:* 31–49, 1968.

7. Kallmann, F. J. The genetic theory of schizophrenia. An analysis of 691 schizophrenic twin index families. Am. J. Psychiatry *103:* 309–322, 1946.
8. Slater, E., with Shields, J. *Psychotic and Neurotic Illnesses in Twins.* Special Report of the Medical Research Council, 278. London, H. M. Stationery Office, 1953.
9. Heston, L. L. Psychiatric disorders in foster home reared children of schizophrenic mothers. Br. J. Psychiatry *112:* 819–825, 1966.
10. Slater, E., Beard, A. W., and Glithero, E. The schizophrenia-like psychoses of epilepsy (I-IV). Br. J. Psychiatry *109:* 95–258, 1963.

7

The antisocial personality and similar disorders

THE CONCEPT OF "PERSONALITY DISORDER"

DSM II defines personality disorder as "characterized by deeply ingrained maladaptive patterns of behavior that are perceptibly different in quality from psychotic and neurotic symptoms. Generally, these are lifelong patterns, often recognizable by the time of adolescence or earlier." [1] The manual then goes on to name 12 such conditions (exclusive of sexual deviation, alcoholism, and drug addiction), briefly describing 10 of them. Some of these labels, for example, "obsessive-compulsive" and "cyclothymic," imply that such patients have mild, chronic varieties or precursors of established syndromes, in these instances obsessive-compulsive neurosis and manic-depressive illness, respectively. Other labels are simply adjectives, purportedly describing key qualities of the personalities in question, for example "asthenic," "inadequate," and "passive-dependent." These labels may eventually prove valid, but as far as we are aware, no studied have yet demonstrated the usefulness of such terminology in predicting outcome or in describing conditions that remain stable over time. By contrast, one personality disorder in DSM II, the antisocial personality, stands as an established syndrome in its own right. "Sociopathy" and "psychopathic personality" also are terms which designate this syndrome.* Notable longitudinal studies establishing the respectability of this as a diagnostic term have been carried out by Robins[2] and the

* The term "hysteria," as defined by Perley and Guze,[4] can now be viewed as an established diagnosis. This might be considered a personality disorder because of its early onset, chronicity, consistency of course over time, behavioral disturbances, and possible kinship to antisocial personality. This last relationship was discovered in family studies, by Guze and his co-workers,[5, 6] who have demonstrated a high incidence of antisocial personality among the male relatives of hysterics, and of hysteria in the female relatives of people with antisocial personality. Guze's diagnosis of hysteria is not used as a diagnosis in DSM II; but the terms "hysterical neurosis" and "hysterical personality" are listed separately, and each only partially describes the syndrome. Such incomplete definition and the double classification of hysteria in DSM II reflect the controversy still surrounding this term.

Gluecks,[3] and other work on this subject has recently been reviewed by Cadoret.[7]

DEFINITION OF ANTISOCIAL PERSONALITY

In her 30-year follow-up study of 524 child guidance clinic patients, Robins[2] described 19 symptoms that were common among the 94 subjects who turned out to have antisocial personalities as adults. According to her criteria, at least five of the 19 symptoms were required for the diagnosis, although the presence of enough symptoms did not automatically make the diagnosis. For example, a subject with mania or schizophrenia might have antisocial symptoms for a time, yet not qualify for the diagnosis, antisocial personality, because the course of the illness and additional symptoms were those of another disorder.

1. Poor work history
2. Poor marital history
3. Excessive drugs
4. Heavy drinking
5. Repeated arrests
6. Physical aggression
7. Sexual promiscuity or perversion
8. Suicide attempts
9. Impulsive behavior
10. School problems and truancy
11. Public financial care
12. Poor armed services record
13. Vagrancy
14. Many somatic symptoms
15. Pathological lying
16. Lack of friends
17. Use of aliases
18. Lack of guilt about sexual exploits and crimes
19. Reckless youth

The above symptoms were common in adult sociopaths. Their disorders began in childhood, and tended to be chronic and resistent to treatment, although 40% had marked diminution of antisocial behavior by their mid-40's. Even the improved sociopath often remained irritable and relatively isolated socially, with continued interpersonal difficulties.

A perusal of Robins' symptom list makes it obvious that adolescents are too young for some symptoms to have occurred, for example, poor job, marital, and armed services histories. In view of this, although we adhered to Robins' general format for diagnosing antisocial personality, our criteria were more lenient than hers. We required only four symptoms instead of five. Our criteria, adapted from those of Robins', follow:

Antisocial Personality: A chronic disorder with at least four of the following symptoms:

1. School problems: recurrent truancy, suspensions or expulsions for misbehavior, fighting
2. Poor work history (if not in school): Firings, quitting jobs with no other jobs available, personality conflicts or fights at work
3. Excessive drug use, with social, scholastic, or work impairment
4. Excessive alcohol use, with social, scholastic, or work impairment

5. Arrests: three or more non-traffic arrests
6. Habitual physical aggressiveness
7. Sexual promiscuity or perversion
8. Suicide attempts
9. Habitually impulsive behavior
10. Vagrancy
11. Many somatic symptoms
12. Habitual lying
13. Few friends
14. Use of aliases (to conceal identity, not as a joke)
15. Lack of guilt

The above list of symptoms gives a clue as to why it has been possible to define antisocial personality more firmly than other personality disorders. These items, except "lack of guilt," are not simply personality characteristics: they describe specific behavior, which can be verified by informants and public records. In addition, however, most observers *would* ascribe certain characteristics to sociopaths: such terms as irritable, selfish, impatient, shallow, cold-hearted, immature, manipulative, irresponsible, and callous are a partial list. It is not unusual for parents and teachers to describe future sociopaths by such adjectives, even before flagrant misbehavior has brought the youngsters into open conflict with social institutions.

PREDICTORS OF ANTISOCIAL BEHAVIOR AND POSSIBLE CAUSES

Future sociopathic behavior can be predicted by childhood antisocial activity such as cruelty, truancy, fighting, lying, and stealing. The more of such behavior the child manifests, the more likely he is to become an antisocial adolescent and adult, regardless of his social class or family structure. In addition, Robins[2] has shown that for a child with such symptoms, certain factors increase his susceptibility for the later development of an antisocial personality. For example, having an antisocial or alcoholic father is a bad prognostic factor. And the lack of firm, consistent discipline and supervision make a sociopathic future more likely for a misbehaving child, regardless of whether or not the father is sociopathic, and regardless of social class.

Although people with antisocial personality are over-represented among the poor and the black, being reared in poverty and dwelling in a ghetto do not predict an antisocial future for a child who shows no early flagrant misbehavior, whose father is not sociopathic, and who receives adequate supervision. The higher incidence of antisocial personality among those in the lower socioeconomic classes may reflect the fact that people with this disorder (whose fathers in turn may have had this disorder) would by virtue of poor job history and criminal behavior naturally tend to drift to, or remain in, the lower classes. But Robins' figures indicate that, given a child with antisocial behavior, being poor and black may increase to some extent his chances of becoming an adult sociopath.[8] Perhaps the stultifying effects of his environment, providing fewer opportunities or rewards for constructive behavior and more incentive for destructive behavior, might operate as independent determinants of an eventual antisocial outcome. This problem, the precise nature of the relationship between social class and delinquency, has been examined by Robins[8] and the Dohrenwends,[9] but no definitive answer has been forthcoming.

Also unanswered is the fundamental question: are there inherited or acquired constitutional factors which render a child susceptible to the restlessness, aggressiveness, etc., which may be precursors of antisocial behavior? Some investigators have suggested that this may at times be the case. For example, in several studies sociopaths have been shown to have a higher proportion of electroencephalographic abnormalities than controls, although there is controversy as to whether any specific patterns of abnormality are correlated with delinquent behavior.[10] Second, recent work by Schulsinger[11] suggests a hereditary factor in that there was a higher incidence of antisocial personality among the biologic relatives of 57 sociopaths adopted early in life than among the biologic relatives of normal adoptees (14.4% *vs.* 6.7%). Third, five studies reviewed by Cadoret[7] demonstrated a greater concordance for sociopathy among monozygotic than dizygotic twins, and the difference was striking in three of these studies. Fourth, Morrison and Stewart,[12] in a family study of hyperkinetic children, found a high incidence of antisocial personality, alcoholism, and hysteria among their parents, and at follow-up into adolescence the children themselves demonstrated an unusual prevalence of antisocial behavior.[13] This last work suggests that the hyperkinetic syndrome, which some investigators blame on minimal brain damage or delayed CNS maturation, may be a precursor of antisocial behavior, and suggests a possible biologic substratum for the disorder in some people.

OTHER PERSONALITY DISORDERS

Among psychiatric patients there is a large group who fit the DSM II description of personality disorder, in that they have "ingrained maladaptive patterns of behavior" which appear by adolescence and are perhaps "life-long," but who are neither sociopaths nor hysterics by our research criteria. As mentioned above, DSM II provides a number of adjectival categories for such people. In Europe, several other classification systems have been constructed to fit these patients. But the classification of the non-sociopathic personality disorders has been even less satisfactory than the various systems in use for classifying neuroses, organic brain syndromes, and the "functional psychoses." In clinical investigations at Washington University, it has been the practice to designate such patients as "undiagnosed." Recently, Liss, Welner, and Robins[14] reviewed 212 consecutive records of discharged inpatients of all ages who had been diagnosed by their own physicians as having some type of personality disorder, exclusive of sociopathy. For example, 39 were "passive-aggressive," 26 "emotionally unstable," 17 "inadequate," 13 "schizoid," and so forth. Of the 212 patients, the investigators were able to reclassify 114 (54%), according to well established syndromes, using strict research criteria. Thirty-seven had depression, 22 were sociopaths, 16 alcoholics, etc. There remained 98 patients still undiagnosed, 94 of whom had too few symptoms for any established diagnostic category. These 94 patients had a mean age of 25, about 15 years younger than the average Renard inpatient. Onset had been at an average age of 19.2 ± 8.3 years. Many of these subjects were described as manipulative, impulsive, and immature, and subject to temper tantrums. Eighty-five percent had marital discord. An extremely high proportion, 51%, had a history of suicide attempts, and in 37% a recent suicide attempt had been the primary reason for hospitalization. In another 17%, the main precipitant of admission had been discord with a spouse or lover.

The investigators followed up 40 of the 94 subjects after an average of four years,[15] 16 (40%) were then classifiable according to established syndromes, but 60% remained "undiagnosed." Thus there is a significant sample of patients, so far not precisely classifiable as antisocial personality or as any other established syndrome, who seem to merit the designation "personality disorder," in that they have the early onset of chronic interpersonal difficulties, and continue to show immaturity, impulsiveness, and manipulativeness. From such longitudinal studies as this, new and distinct types of personality disorder may emerge as clear-cut syndromes and become established as respectable diagnoses with consistent clinical pictures and courses over time.

ADOLESCENTS IN THE STUDY WITH ANTISOCIAL PESONALITY

The Distinctness of Antisocial Personality from Other Established Syndromes

The teenagers in our study with antisocial personality differed from those with other established syndromes in several respects. First, their disorders were characterized principally by antagonistic and non-conforming (not bizarre) behavior, which brought them into conflict with their schools and families. There was also a notable absence of disorders of the form and content of thought, or of serious affective disturbance: the quality of "depression" in the 40% of the sociopaths who complained of it (see Table 33, below) was comparatively shallow and often seemed simply a reaction to the frustrating circumstances which their own behavior had brought about.

Second, unlike other psychiatric inpatients, the antisocial adolescents seemed to cause more suffering in other people than they experienced themselves. As a consequence, by the time the patients entered this study they had encountered a good deal of social rejection, but a case can not be made that they were initially rejected by their parents (although, as mentioned above, actual deprivation of a parent was not unusual). On the contrary, despite the interpersonal conflicts that raged in their homes, the parents' behavior toward their children was characterized by repeated attempts to help them mature, to find the right schools, the right camps, the right therapists, and so forth. As these attempts were recurrently frustrated, the parents often reacted with demandingness, anger, and

TABLE 33

Common Symptoms among Adolescents with Antisocial Personality and "Undiagnosed, Most Like Antisocial Personality"

N = 20

	Girls N = 10	Boys N = 10	Total N = 20
	%	%	%
Alcohol use*	70	90	80
Ever expelled or suspended from school for misbehavior	50	80	65
Truant more than once a year	60	70	65
Arguing	80	40	60
Arrested, ever	50	50	50
Sexual intercourse, ever	20	80	50
Nervousness	50	50	50
Temper outbursts	70	30	50
Running away overnight	50	40	45
Stealing	40	50	45
In trouble at school for fighting	40	50	45
History of head injury	30	60	45
Too old for grade	50	30	40
Depressed	40	40	40
Percentage of parents toward whom patients felt negative†	28	40	35
Suicidal thoughts‡	50	20	35
Decreased interest	40	30	35
Ever held back academically	30	30	30
Insomnia	40	20	30

* Three girls and two boys (25%) had a history of excessive alcohol use or regular use at an inappropriately early age (*e.g.*, 12).

† Assessment of attitudes toward the 37 current functional parents.

‡ One boy and three girls (20%) *attempted* suicide.

grief; but we were impressed that, in the main, the mothers and fathers had withstood a great deal of provocation and persisted in sincere efforts to be primarily helpful, rather than primarily punitive. The antisocial children, compared with their siblings, had absorbed far more than their share of the families' money and attention, responding in general with neither gratitude nor improvement. Of course, as previously mentioned, these antisocial adolescents were a special group, perhaps differing from the general population of sociopaths in some essential respects. By virtue of the fact that they were selected from inpatients in a private hospital, the odds were high that they would be found to have families who were primarily trying to help them.

A third major difference between the antisocial group and most of the patients with other established syndromes lay in their lack of response to the conventional modes of treatment. For this reason, the sociopaths were typically very frustrating for psychiatrists and other therapists to work with. The doctor could not push a button on an ECT machine or administer medication and alter such a patient's pattern of misbehavior; nor did the patients themselves usually have or acquire the motivation to pursue a course of psychotherapy or behavior modification. Sociopaths at times entered treatment with superficial motivation, but usually lost it when sustained initiative and internal discipline was required of them. They usually did not see themselves as needing to change very much, but rather as needing fewer social restrictions. Furthermore, they often lacked the capacity to form a sufficiently productive relationship with their therapists, which could have served to enhance whatever motivation to change they did possess.

Our teenagers with antisocial personality were thus notably resistant to change, whether treatment was in the context of the medical model or the social model or a combination of the two. It followed that hospitalization of such patients on the ordinary psychiatric inpatient unit could not be considered adequate treatment of the underlying condition. The physicians admitting our sociopathic teenagers to Renard Hospital knew this, and admission was usually recommended (or forced) to cope with temporarily disruptive behavior and to relieve social pressure, with no expectation that the hospital stay would provide definitive treatment or long-term benefit. The hospital was more often a "way station" on a long road—a temporary expedient to deal with yet another crisis in a long series of difficulties. The ultimate solution, or the process which would hopefully lead to improvement, lay in establishing the teenagers in other settings (at home or in schools, for example) and pursuing therapeutic approaches other than placement in an expensive acute inpatient treatment center.

General Characteristics of Antisocial Patients in the Study

There were ten adolescents (seven psychiatric inpatients and three controls) who qualified for the diagnosis, antisocial personality, by our criteria and another 10 (also seven patients and three controls) who failed to qualify only because they had too few antisocial symptoms. The latter ten were designated "undiagnosed, most like antisocial personality." The two groups did not differ from each other with respect to type of clinical picture, family history, age of onset, current age, sex distribution, or the number of symptoms exclusive of antisocial symptoms, for example, depression, suicide attempts, and somatic complaints. Thus the "undiagnosed" group with primary behavior disorder seemed to be mildly disturbed sociopaths, and we believe it would be splitting hairs to present them here as a separate group. They may, of course, later develop some other (as yet undefined) type of personality disorder, or have a higher rate of remission than sociopaths with more symptoms. But because of the similar quality of their clinical picture, all 20 subjects are considered as a group in this chapter.

In reviewing these data the reader should remember that, although these 20 subjects might be considered typical of a group of antisocial adolescents admitted to a private psychiatric and medical facility (only 16 other teenagers were discharged from Renard with the diagnosis, antisocial personality, during the study period), no claim can be made that this group is representative of youthful sociopaths in the general population. Most young sociopaths do not receive inpatient psychiatric care. Many are referred for outpatient psychiatric evaluation and treatment, especially if they are middle-class whites; and many others, especially the poor and the black, may simply be handled by law enforcement agencies and pass through juvenile courts. Factors which result in an antisocial teenager's being admitted to a psychiatric hospital are such things as having parents or guardians who are able and willing to pay for hospitalization, making suicide attempts or threats, and having other psychiatric symptoms, such as depression or anxiety, which initially may lead physicians to believe that the patients have other psychiatric disorders more amenable to short-term hospital treatment than antisocial personality.

Of the 20 patients considered in this chapter, ten were boys and ten were girls. Two patients were black, 17 white, and one an American Indian. They ranged in age from 12 to 19 (mean 16.0), and at the time of admission the girls were, on the average, younger than the boys (15.6 years and 16.4 years, respectively). Only four of the 20 adolescent sociopaths had been in a psychiatric hospital prior to the study admission, but the average patient had been impaired by the symptoms leading to hospitalization for three and a half years, since age 12½. However, troublesome character traits had often begun in early childhood and had not become manifest as flagrant misbehavior until around puberty, or shortly before.

Family and Social Backgrounds

As a group, the antisocial teenagers were of lower socioeconomic status than the total sample of subjects in our study. Thirty percent of them came from families earning more than $10,000 a year *vs.* 48% of our other teenagers. The mean socioeconomic index was 33 for antisocial psychiatric inpatients, 26 for antisocial controls (*vs.* 48 and 40, respectively, for all patients and controls). Half the family wage earners worked below the skilled level, as compared with only a quarter of the wage earners of families of non-sociopaths. All previous publications on antisocial personality led us to expect these findings.

Despite the relatively lower social status of the antisocial teenagers, however, they were not a destitute group. They were, after all, patients in a private hospital. Half the wage-earning parents were in skilled, white collar, or executive positions, and 40% were above the average socioeconomic index of the total study sample. Moreover, for the 13 teenagers tested, I.Q.'s ranged from 85 to 136 with a median of 103, and a mean of 105. Thus our modal antisocial teenager was middle class and of normal intelligence, giving us the opportunity to study this syndrome in somewhat more "privileged" young sociopaths than most found in the general population.

The family backgrounds were significantly more chaotic than those of non-sociopaths. In 55% of the cases, at least one natural parent was absent from the home, compared to only 28% of the teenagers without antisocial personality. Of the 20 adolescents, four had experienced parental divorce, one was born out of wedlock, and six, 30%, had lost parents through death (two mothers, four fathers). By contrast only 7% of the non-sociopathic adolescents had a dead parent ($p < 0.001$). Four of the parental deaths were from heart disease or cancer. A fifth lost her mother in an automobile accident with no evidence that the accident was related to alcohol abuse or other antisocial activity. The sixth death was in an alcoholic father who committed suicide when the patient was ten, four years before his admission to this study.

The incidence of parental divorce or separation was the same among sociopaths as among all other study subjects (20% and 21%, respectively). With respect to broken homes, then, it was really the high incidence of parental death which distinguished sociopathic adolescents from the non-sociopaths. The deaths of the parents had had a marked and long-lasting emotional effect on at least three of the six bereaved children. They and their surviving parents dated the onset of antisocial activity immediately after the fathers' deaths when the patients were, respectively, eight, ten, and 13 years of age. Misbehavior had then continued for ten, four, and seven years, respectively. The boy who had been ten years old when his father committed suicide had continued to ruminate about the death during the four intervening years. No direct influence on the course of sociopathy could be demonstrated in the other three bereaved teenagers. But it is notable that all four of the sociopaths who had made suicide attempts had lost parents through death. However, the suicide attempts were not temporally associated with the parents' deaths (the shortest interval was four years), and the boy whose alcoholic father had killed himself was not a suicide attempter.

The 20 sociopaths came from families of the same size as the 200 non-sociopathic subjects of this study. The incidence of parental psychopathology was higher than among parents of other psychiatrically ill teenagers: 55% of the sociopaths had ill parents. Six of the 20 fathers (30%) were alcoholic, one was depressed. Three mothers (15%) had depression, and one was schizophrenic. Antisocial personality was not found among the parents of these subjects. Thus the pattern of psychopathology among the sick parents of sociopaths was distinguished principally by a high incidence of alcoholism among the fathers. There were five psychiatrically ill siblings: one alcoholic, one sociopath, and three "undiagnosed." Incidence figures mean little with respect to siblings, most of whom were still teenagers or children.

The Clinical Picture and Course of Antisocial Personality

Table 33 shows the symptoms most frequently found in the 20 antisocial teenagers. This list is markedly different from those for patients with affective disorders, schizophrenia, and schizoaffective illness. Among other things, the symptoms of sociopathy reflected a characteristic that set these teenagers apart from those who were psychiatrically well or who had other established syndromes: their behavior was precociously venturesome. They were early risk-takers who dared at a young age to enter into activity which, according to standard codes of conduct, should have been reserved for the late teens or adulthood. In addition, of course, they engaged in behavior that would have been considered socially unacceptable at any age. They began to drink, smoke, engage in sexual activity, drive cars, and absent themselves from home in the evenings much sooner than other, less daring adolescents, although not necessarily sooner than those other adolescents wanted to do these things. Unfortunately, along with this prospensity to rush into the "adult pleasures" of tobacco, alcohol, sex, driving, and freedom from parental restraint, there was a notable lack of the sense of responsibility and inner restraints that keep such behavior in bounds. Despite their social precocity, these teenagers were immature and irresponsible compared to their normal peers.

Their precocity may be a reflection of the physical and emotional restlessness, and the inability to stay in one place or stick to expected tasks, that often characterized the future sociopaths early in their childhoods. This restlessness often overrode all attempts, however ingenious, of parents and teachers to check it or channel it into socially acceptable, conforming behavior. Perhaps the significantly higher rate of parental death in this group contributed to a relative lessening of discipline and domestic stability which these patients may have needed more than most children do. Perhaps, too, the higher rate of alcoholism in their fathers played a causative role in their own early drinking, either through genetic means, or social modeling, or a combination of both factors. But all statements about cause in this particular group of sociopaths are speculative.

Designation of onset could not be precise for a disorder in which childhood impulsiveness, aggressivity, and other traits often preceded flagrant misbehavior by several years. These personality characteristics may be the essence of the disorder, and perhaps its onset should be scored with their first appearance. But most rambunctious, difficult, or hyperactive children do not become sociopaths, so there appears to be no certain way of designating the beginning of the disorder except by the appearance of overtly antisocial acts which impaired a child at home and school. Judged by this standard, onset in our group ranged from ages nine to 16, with an average of 12.43 years and a median age of 13. The mean age of onset was not significantly different for girls than for boys (12.56 and 12.30 years, respectively), although the girls were younger at the time of the study. They entered the hospital an average of 3.0 years after the beginning of antisocial symptoms; the boys entered 4.1 years after onset. The greater prevalence of suicidal threats and attempts among sociopathic girls might have been a factor bringing about their earlier hospitalization.

As seen in Table 33, alcohol use was the most common symptom, and was present in all but one boy and three girls. Only 25% had a history of excessive or inappropriate alcohol use, but this proportion might be expected to increase with age: the average patient was 16. Illegal drug use was less common, with only 30% of the patients admitting to it. This may have increased in St. Louis teenagers since the time of this study.

School was a prominent site of difficulty. Two-thirds had significant truancy, and two-thirds had been expelled or suspended for bad behavior at least once. Almost half had been in trouble for fighting, and almost one-third had been held back at least once for academic reasons. Forty percent had been a year or more too old for their school grade at some time in their scholastic careers.

Typically the first year of academic failure was at age eight or nine, in primary school (average, 4th grade), whereas trouble with fights began at ages 10 to 12 (average, 6th grade), and both truancy and suspension for misbehavior first occurred at ages 12 to 14 (average, 8th grade). At the time of the study, five patients (25%) had dropped out of school. This occurred during high school for 80% of the drop-outs. Thus academic problems were typically manifested early and were a reflection of inattention, restlessness, and underachievement, rather than of low intelligence. Significant belligerence in school and truancy occurred later.

Trouble at home and in the community were evident by the high proportion who were markedly argumentative (60%), had temper tantrums (50%), ran away overnight (45%), and were arrested by the police (50%). The degree of conflict engendered by their behavior and their families' hostility is evident in the high proportion of parents toward whom the sociopaths had almost exclusively negative feelings, not even mixed with positive feelings. The 20 teenagers had 37 currently functional parents (including step or foster parents). Predominantly negative feelings were expressed concerning 35% of these parents. The 200 study subjects who were not sociopathic felt mainly negative about only 18% of their 383 current parents ($p < 0.05$).

Sociopaths had no history of prenatal difficulties or neonatal illness and injury. Although 45% of them had a history of head injury, only two had had this trauma before their antisocial behavior began; another patient had a febrile illness with unconsciousness early in childhood. In no instances were there sequelae which suggested that brain injury might have played a causative role in onset of sociopathy, although one boy had an increase in antisocial behavior after a head injury. Injuries were more typically the results of their daring behavior, rather than the cause of their lack of inner control.

The standard symptoms of severe mood and thought disorder so common among our other ill subjects were rarer among sociopaths. Subjective nervousness, present in 50% of the sociopaths, was a leading symptom and was a reflection of their restlessness and impatience. Depressive feelings (40%) were typically related to frustrating situations and were short-lived. Suicidal thoughts and attempts were less prominent than among the psychiatrically ill teenagers with other diagnoses. Somatic complaints were not prominent—20% had headaches, 25% nausea, 25% back pain.

Eight of the ten boys and only two of the ten girls admitted to sexual intercourse. (The boys were, on the average, nearly a year older than the girls.) All antisocial subjects who had sexual experience had done so at age 16 or earlier. The first experience was typically at age 14 or 15. As young as these subjects were, 60% of them had "gone steady" or been engaged at least once, compared to 40% of non-sociopathic study subjects, who were a mean of seven months older than the sociopaths. No subject admitted to homosexual activity.

Boys and girls differed little as to the clinical picture, except that more girls had temper outbursts, argumentativeness, and suicidal thoughts and attempts; the boys were more sexually precocious and had a higher incidence of head injuries.

Hospitalization of the Antisocial Teenager: Precipitating Factors and Goals

Only four of the 14 psychiatric inpatients with antisocial personality (the controls were hospitalized on medical-surigcal services for reasons other than their psychiatric disorder) had had prior psychiatric hospitalizations. All these had been brief. During the study admission, the psychiatric patients were in the hospital from 4 to 122 days, with an average stay of 26 days and a median of 14 days. If the patient with the longest stay is eliminated from calculation, the mean length of hospitalization was only 18 days. Only two patients received antidepressants, one a tranquilizer, another an anticonvulsant. No one was given ECT. The typical treatment was psychotherapy and the restraint and social control of being in the hospital. There was no real evidence that these patients were fundamentally different when they were discharged from the way they had been when they were admitted. Most were poorly motivated, vexatious, and manipulative while they were hospitalized. In a disorder such as this, with questionable benefit derived from hospitalization itself, it is important for us to examine the reasons why these patients were admitted, and the goals of hospitalization from the points of view of patients, families, and physicians.

Table 34 lists the immediate causes for hospitalization of the 20 teenagers with antisocial personality. Five (84%) of the six controls (from non-psychiatric wards) had been admitted for treatment of trauma; only 13% of non-sociopathic controls were in the hospital as a result of trauma ($p <$ 0.001). Moreover, the trauma was the direct result of antisocial activity in four of the five injured controls. The only control who was not admitted because of injury (C-076) had developed abdominal pain while drinking. The hospitalization of the six antisocial controls on medical and surgical services was not related to treatment for personality disorder as such. Those patients had never been hospitalized for treatment of psychiatric conditions.

The 14 sociopaths who were psychiatric inpatients presented a more

TABLE 34

Immediate Precipitants of Hospital Admission for 20 Adolescents with Antisocial Personality

Psychiatric Inpatients

Code	Age	Race	Sex	Reason for Admission
Y-018	16	W	M	Intoxicated from glue-sniffing
Y-023	15	W	F	Wrecked car while driving illegally
Y-036	12	W	F	Refused to go to school
Y-037	14	W	M	Truancy and glue-sniffing
Y-043	18	AI	F	Drunk and fighting
Y-054	16	W	M	Ran away, returned, had arguments with father
Y-055	17	W	F	Ran away
Y-062	15	W	F	Jilted by boy, suicide threat
Y-065	18	W	F	Hallucinations due to drugs
Y-069	18	W	F	Threatened suicide
Y-072	19	W	M	Just released from jail for robbery. Judge advised hospital because of prior head injury
Y-080	19	W	M	Narcotics agent gave choice of hospital or prosecution
Y-086	12	B	M	Kicked teacher
Y-093	14	W	F	Threatened to kill mother and self

Controls (On Nonpsychiatric Services)

Code	Age	Race	Sex	Reason for Admission
C-010	16	W	F	Shot in chest by common-law husband because of promiscuity
C-013	16	W	M	Driving too fast, lost control, fractured mandible
C-015	13	B	F	Knocked out in fight
C-076	19	W	M	Acute onset of abdominal pain while drinking
C-103	16	W	M	Bomb he was making exploded in his hand
C-107	17	W	M	Gasoline caught fire while he was cleaning with it

complicated picture from the standpoint of over-all motivation for hospitalization. In general, the immediate reasons for admission were merely incidental. These adolescents were put into a psychiatric facility in the hope (by themselves, parents, or doctors) that treatment there would begin the process of changing the direction of lives that had gone awry some time before.

As to the immediate precipitants of hospitalization, three of the 14 sociopaths in Renard Hospital were admitted for symptoms which required inpatient psychiatric observation to guard against self-destructiveness and rule out treatable affective disorder. These were patients Y-062, Y-069, and Y-093, who had threatened suicide. For the other 11 antisocial psychiatric inpatients, the immediate precipitants of admission were typical antisocial acts, in no way uncharacteristic of their past behavior.

Although all 11 of these teenagers were believed to need temporary external control in some sort of institution, only for three, who were acutely intoxicated at the time of admission (Y-018, Y-043, and Y-065), was it ideal that this control be in a psychiatric hospital rather than some other type of place.

In all 14 cases of sociopaths in the psychiatric hospital, the immediate problems precipitating admission were alleviated within a matter of days. Such behavior as suicidal threats, drug taking, drinking, running away, and fighting were brought to a temporary halt, and absence from school became sanctioned, since the patients were in a hospital under psychiatric treatment. But everyone involved with these patients, including the patients themselves, knew or suspected that hospitalization would bring only transient cessation of the problems. These adolescents were motivated poorly, or not at all, to change, and the parents knew from experience that their hopes had been raised on many previous occasions (as they transferred their children from school to school, or from doctor to doctor), only to be dashed by the recurrence of antisocial behavior. As judged by their behavior during the study admission, the short-term outcome of hospitalization in Renard proved to be no different from previous attempts to set these patients going in a more productive direction. Only follow-up will reveal whether some of the teenagers later enter long-term treatment or school situations that will be conducive to change, whether their antisocial behavior will remit spontaneously, or worsen.

Five typical cases are reported here.

> Y-018—This 16-year-old white boy was admitted after he became intoxicated from sniffing glue.
>
> There was no history of psychopathology in the immediate family, nor of parental deprivation. His father was a skilled laborer. The boy was described as "restless, nervous, and fidgety since the time he was born." The only significant childhood illness was measles, with a high fever and delirium, at age four. In first grade (age six) his behavior suddenly changed "as if it weren't him": he would fail to complete tasks, leave his things around, be inattentive and restless, and get into fights. A neurologic evaluation at age eight produced no significant findings. School problems continued and, along with his general behavior, worsened at the time of puberty, though he stopped fighting after elementary school. At age 13 the school described him as follows: "highly nervous, classroom disturbances and family problems of a nature. He was thin . . . and much aware of his physical weakness. He was wise to teachers. He would go along okay for awhile and appear to have an emotional upset and then have weeks of problems at school" "He was a mixed-up boy, unable to adapt to our school program . . . received a great deal of attention

here, and teachers tried to work with him." He began to fail subjects routinely. During the ninth grade (age 14) more serious trouble began. He clowned in the classrooms, argued with teachers, and refused to work. His teacher wrote: "____ is not a mean boy. He just hasn't grown up yet. He finds so many little things to do to amuse himself. He just doesn't let himself be bothered about studies and adjusting to school schedule. He is pleasant and doesn't resent being disciplined, but he has forgotten it in five minutes. He is constantly trying to draw some student's attention to himself. You think you have him busy, and the minute you turn your back he is either tripping someone or doing some other disturbing thing." He was expelled from school at the end of the 9th grade. At about this time his grooming became poor, and for a few months he had a head-shaking tic.

At age 15, he began to have overt conflict with his parents and to become arrogant and really unmanageable at home for the first time. He was accordingly placed in a small residential treatment center, where he remained for the 18 months prior to admission, and where his behavior continued to worsen. He was arrested on four occasions: for shoplifting, vandalism, threatening the staff, and car theft during his stay there, age 15 to 16. While at this treatment center he became intimate with another student, a 16-year-old girl. They had sexual relations on a regular basis, and two months before the patient's admission to Renard, they ran away from the treatment center together, after which they were both expelled.

Then followed several weeks at home, during which time the patient was idle and became more involved in arguments with his mother, demanding that she leave the house. His girlfriend began to avoid him, frightened of his behavior. He ran away from home. Finally, ruminating over "being pushed around for two years," he took an overdose of sleeping pills while at a friend's house a week prior to admission at Renard. He was treated in the St. Louis City Hospital emergency room and released. His parents then arranged for him to live with an uncle, where, during the five days before admission, he sniffed glue. He entered Renard Hospital after being picked up in an inebriated state from the effects of those fumes.

Upon admission the mother said he was irresponsible, uncontrollable, and had been dissatisfied since school troubles began almost three years before. The patient said he "just had depression. I had no place to go. I just grew up too fast in the time at Methodist Children's Home." During the hospital stay he broke rules frequently and became hostile whenever his immediate demands were not met. He socialized poorly, but depression was not a problem.

Y-054—The mother of this 16-year-old white boy expressed her son's problem, and that of many others like him, most succinctly as she spoke to the admitting psychiatrist: "He doesn't want to go to school; he felt in a cage at school. But he can't cope with being *out* of school and can't get a job. He is very belligerent at home and has no communication with us."

His parents were psychiatrically healthy, and caring; but great antagonism had grown up between the boy and his father by his midteens on account of the child's behavior. The patient and his parents dated his difficulties back to age 13. But an elementary school teacher had written, "I have personally known ____ from about 4th grade . . . I have seen him on the verge of difficulty a number of times. He had a tendency to get with wrong companions, was on the point of rebellion at times, and showed signs of temper. At 7th grade I had hopes that he would stabilize as there was definite effort on part of parents to help him; and he showed evidence of their influence."

Those hopes were not to be realized. When he was in 8th grade (age 13), the family moved to an urban area. Although theretofore a tractable person, he then began to run around with boys who were wild, threw rocks at cars, and harrassed people. He began to urge his parents to let him stay out late on school nights and sleep late in the mornings. Conflicts arose over this, his mode of dress, and his negligence of homework. The patient violated his restrictions, and his parents responded chiefly by not speaking to him, or by making him sit still for long hours. He began to be defiant toward his father as restrictions upon him increased. At school he began to fight and liked to identify with the tough crowd. His academic productivity began dropping in eighth grade.

More overt school problems began when he was 14, in ninth grade. He began to feel nervous, unable to concentrate, and to have abdominal bloating and loose stools up to five times a day. He increasingly worried about this, and said that the problem made him want to avoid school. Along with his friends he began to smoke, drink heavily (15 beers in three hours at times), and stay out later at night when he was 14. During that year he and his friends developed a bicycle-theft racket, in which they would alter the serial numbers, repaint the bikes, and sell them. This continued for one year and terminated with the patient's arrest for riding a stolen bicycle; but the extent of the racket was never revealed to the police, and the patient was merely reprimanded. He also indulged in vandalism during this time.

In 10th grade this illegal behavior diminished, but the boy's conflicts with his family increased. He would spend nights away from home and absent himself from school, pleading illness as an excuse. From age 15 until his admission, one year later, he was increasingly demanding and rude to his parents, and about once or twice a week had temper outbursts, threw things, and made threats. Despite all this, his father bought him an old car when he became 16 years old, which the patient had wanted to work on and fix up himself. But he took no initiative in this matter.

At the start of 11th grade he felt "too cooped up" to stay in school, and would not go. His father, refusing to "harbor a drop-out," had the car towed away and insisted he move out. He stayed for a few days with his grandparents, then he and two friends left for California in an automobile. They were picked up by police in Kansas City. The patient was returned home, where he continued to be quarrelsome and defiant. At this point he was admitted to Renard. There had never been a history of drug use, but occasional heavy drinking had continued.

His psychiatrist hoped to begin the process of outpatient therapy after brief hospitalization, and the boy's attitude at first seemed promising. But after discharge he refused to go with his parents for office visits.

Y-055—This white girl was 17 years old upon admission. She and her parents gave a history of behavioral difficulty dating back to age 14. Yet the school reports which were collected during our study revealed problems dating back to first grade (age six). While the child was in early primary school, teachers (and the mother herself) were disposed to blame the parents or at least to transfer to them the responsibility for doing something about the situation at school. The following statements by teachers are illustrative: "(The mother) said perhaps she herself was making the child nervous or jittery over success at school by pushing her at home . . . ____'s worst habit is inattention and talking with others during work periods (age 6)." "____ appears pale and frightened in my judgment . . . ____ talks too much and too often . . . good disposition, friendly, likes to help out . . . trouble getting along with the other children and with me. She has gotten in other children's desks and storied to me a number of times (age eight)." This and other reports show that a picture was already beginning to develop of an overly active, verbose child who could be charming as well as devious and truculent. From age eight to ten the school transferred much of the responsbility for schoolwork onto the parents, and quotes from the child indicated that by age nine she was adept at shifting the blame for her nervousness to her parents. The teachers seemed to accept this on slender evidence, for example, on the basis of the mother's reacting defensively at being blamed for her child's over-talkativeness and short attention span. However, by the time the patient was in 9th grade (age 14), teachers' reports concentrated merely on her own behavior, which had not changed in character: "Impatience, short attention span." "____ has failed every test . . . she just was not studying at all and did not care about her grade . . . doesn't pay attention . . . needs to be calmed down and come to school prepared to concentrate." Prodding would occasionally bring improvement, then she would revert to form when the pressure was off.

More overt conflict with her mother and the school began between ages 13 and 15, as the patient pushed for increasingly liberal social privileges and gravitated toward a group of "faster, cheaper, tougher, wilder" girls. When she was 14, she was suspended from school once for smoking, once for having pornographic pictures, was arrested once for shoplifting, and caught for phoning in a false fire alarm and making an anonymous fire-threat to the school. By age 14, she was lying casually, without the motive to cover misdeeds. Her school grades had dropped by age 15, and her interest in athletics, a former area of high achievement, waned also. Her failure to complete tasks or follow through on activities requiring discipline became more marked. She gained weight excessively, once she lost interest in athletics. Although she made friends rapidly, she had trouble holding on to them because of her unreliability and her tendency to shift blame to others. As for dating, she insisted that a boy "kiss my feet" before she would consider going out with him.

At age 16, seven months before admission, she ran away from home for the first time. This was an impulsive act to accompany two older boys who had been quarreling with their parents. The trio stayed with a relative of one of the boys for three days, then were returned in police custody. Her parents had had no warning of the absence, nor was it directly related to stress at home. During the seven months before her Renard admission, she was increasingly defiant at home, refusing to do her chores, having temper outbursts, and lying. She told people untruths about her parents: that they beat her, bought clothes extravagantly, and that her mother was a drunkard and sexually promiscuous.

Four months before admission she left home again and did not return, living with various friends despite her parents' pleas and legal efforts to get her back home. Her grandparents refused to let her stay with them because of her defiant and devious behavior after a few days there. Thereafter she refused to keep her parents advised as to her whereabouts. On one occasion during this four-month period she and another girl spent $900 of the latter's savings in a few days while in a motel. There was an unknown amount of involvement with men at this time. On another occasion she drank "16 shots" of whisky in 15 minutes "on a dare" from friends, who abandoned her in a car in a roadside ditch when she passed out. She was taken to the St. Louis County Hospital by a passing motorist and spent seven days on their psychiatric ward. Her admission to Renard Hospital was six weeks later, after she truanted from school and was picked up by her parents at a local hamburger stand.

On admission she was cheerful and initially cooperative, but became impatient as the interview progressed. She did not change during her brief hospitalization, nor during a readmission to Renard three weeks after discharge. The family did not follow through on advice to place her in a residential treatment center.

Y-065—This white girl was 18 years old at the time of her admission to Renard Hospital. Her parents were separated when she was three months old because her father was "lazy and sorry" and would not support the family. The child was impulsive, irritable, and "the jealous type" from an early age, and would do things to get revenge on others. From age four until about 14, she had temper tantrums up to twice a month, during which she destroyed objects. When the patient was nine years old, her mother, who had been paralyzed two years previously in an accident, died. Her maternal grandmother reported that the child had a marked emotional reaction to this, and often talked about how good her mother had been. She was subsequently raised by her grandmother. The patient herself, although of normal intelligence, said she remembered little of her life during the four years between her mother's death and age 13.

Her temper tantrums became worse at age ten. By age 13 she began to neglect her schoolwork, but this was not reflected in failing grades until 9th grade, age 14 to 15. By that year she began to be truant from school and to stay out late at night. This was too much for the grandmother to handle, and she was sent to live with her older sister.

She became sexually active at age 16, stating that her first experience was "rape" by a family friend. In the course of the next two years, she had approximately 60 different partners, and was usually orgasmic. At some point during this time, her 23-year-old brother had sexual relations with her. On another occasion, she had intercourse with five boys in quick succession. She stated that both those occurrences were against her will.

By the time of her 17th birthday, her life had become quite chaotic. During the year and a half preceding her admission to

Renard, she was jailed twice for car theft, once for breaking probation, and was confined (for two months at age 17) in a Georgia State Hospital for her behavior disorder. She complained increasingly of restlessness and nervousness and took various tranquilizers during the 18 months prior to entry into Renard. During the six months prior to her 18th birthday she drank heavily, up to two fifths of bourbon daily, although she did not abuse drugs. She traveled about, living in turn with a cousin, a brother, and a sister. At age 18, she made three or four suicide attempts in a period of two months, with tranquilizer overdoses and wrist scratches. These attempts were apparently precipitated by conflicts with a boyfriend, who had beaten her up for being unfaithful to him. Finally, at the age of 18, her antisocial behavior led her relatives to have her confined by a sheriff in Florida for "incompetency." It was decided to enroll her in the Job Corps, and she was assigned to the St. Louis unit of that organization two months before her admission to Renard Hospital. At the Job Corps she was in a dormitory with a number of girls who had had behavior problems. The girls attended high school classes and had vocational training, which in the patient's case was projected to last for 18 months. She remained relatively quiet for the first month in the Job Corps, but during the month before admission she had several absences without leave from the dormitory. She impulsively became "engaged" to a boy she had just met and ran away with him for a few days. Two nights before admission to Renard she took an unknown amount of an over-the-counter medicine containing scopolamine, ostensibly to help her sleep. The police picked her up, the Job Corps personnel locked her in a room. During the next two nights she experienced frightening auditory and visual hallucinations, "saw" and "heard" people walking through the closed door, then fading away, "saw" a man stabbing a woman. She pried loose a bar from her bed and broke the window in order to escape from these imagined dangers. Accordingly, she was sedated and admitted to Renard Hospital.

After her admission she became fully alert and was free of the visions and voices. Her mental status was unremarkable during her brief hospitalization, after which she was discharged from the Job Corps and returned to her home state.

Y-072—This white son of a skilled laborer was 19 years old when he entered Renard Hospital. His admission was arranged by his parents and a judge for psychiatric and neurologic evaluation. He arrived four hours after his release from a 27-day jail term for breaking and entering. The patient stated that the indirect reason for his admission was a need for job training: "I'm mixed up. Got too many scars on me. Can't get a job because they ask: what is this or that scar for?"

The patient's father at first declared that his son had had no problems prior to a head injury sustained in an automobile accident 16 months before admission. The boy was receiving financial compensation from the accident, and his most flagrant antisocial acts had followed it. But the patient himself dated school trouble and fighting back to the primary grades. He had never done well in school. In addition, from age 10 to 14 he had many fights with other boys. He stated that he seldom started the conflicts, but that other boys picked on him because of his reputation as a good fighter. He failed sixth grade (age 11) because of low achievement. The seventh grade was marked by failure in a subject, at least one fist fight with a teacher, and suspension for truancy and smoking. During the eighth grade this behavior intensified, and after several more suspensions he was permanently expelled at age 16.

Serious trouble at home also began at age 16 when his father had him picked up by the police for car theft. In that year he was first knocked unconscious in a fight with other boys. Conflicts with his parents when he was 16 resulted in his brief dismissal from the home, an event that occurred two or three times more in the succeeding three years.

The patient's first serious head injury occurred at age 17 when he was running at a swimming pool and fell. He was unconscious for two hours, then awoke, became wild, and experienced episodes of vomiting. Brief hospitalization for observation resulted in recovery. But one month later (16 months before admission to Renard) he was in a serious automobile accident while in a race with another car. Craniotomy was required for evacuation of subdural and intracerebral hematomas. Postoperatively there was an expressive aphasia which improved (but which was present to a moderate degree at the time of his entry of this study).

Subsequently he had trouble when applying for jobs because of his neurologic deficit. About six months after the automobile accident he was knocked unconscious once more when the transmission of a car he was working under fell on his head.

Shortly thereafter he began staying out later at night, and began to ruminate about his desire to kill another boy who had allegedly been responsible for the patient's younger brother being sent to a juvenile correctional institution. He began to carry a gun at times. At this time he was once more knocked out in a fight.

During the five months prior to his admission to Renard Hospital, his troubles with the law increased. In association with other youths he broke into houses on at least three occasions in a small town near St. Louis. During this period he stayed with his sister and her husband for a time, and on one occasion pointed a pistol at his own neck when frustrated by his sister's attempts to prevent his going to a rough place with other boys.

Police finally caught and jailed him for one month during an episode of breaking and entering a club house. After the month in jail the patient was released by the judge upon appeal from his father, who requested neurologic evaluation concerning the effect of the head injuries on his behavior.

During his hospitalization the boy behaved in exemplary fashion, was cooperative and friendly. He had expressive aphasia, mildly depressed feelings, and moderately slurred speech. Vocational rehabilitation was arranged for the post discharge period.

SUMMARY

Antisocial Personality in the Hospitalized Adolescent

The antisocial personality has been firmly established as a specific syndrome by excellent longitudinal and family studies. It is a chronic disturbance which usually begins in childhood or early adolescence and is marked by behavior which leads to serious difficulties in interpersonal relationships, school problems, and conflicts with legal authorities. Sociopaths are often described as aggressive, impulsive, hyperactive, and demanding, and these traits may be present early in childhood, before flagrant antisocial behavior begins. The disorder is considered resistant to standard forms of psychiatric treatment. It is further complicated by the consequences of school failure, jail terms, alcohol abuse, and so forth, which sociopaths experience. Sociopaths often lead unproductive lives and may spend significant periods of their adult lives in public financial care—in prison, on welfare, etc. In addition, they are often socially isolated by their behavior and by a relative shallowness of their interpersonal relationships.

The causes of this personality disorder are not known. A history of childhood or adolescent antisocial activity is invariably found in adult sociopaths, and is thus a necessary precursor. Some preliminary data suggest a genetic basis for this disorder. In addition, it has been demonstrated that lack of early discipline and supervision predispose some children to sociopathy if they are already behaving badly. Studies have also shown that having a father with alcoholism or sociopathy is an important factor in predicting an eventual antisocial outcome for a child who already has a behavior problem. The role of social class in the genesis of this disturbance is still unclear.

This chapter reviews the data concerning 20 adolescents who had antisocial personalities of varying degrees of severity. They were perhaps typical of adolescent sociopaths in private psychiatric hospitals, and were, in general, Caucasian, of normal intelligence, and from middle income families. Compared to our other study subjects, a significantly greater number of sociopaths, 55%, had experienced some type of parental deprivation, with 30% having lost the parent through death. Loss of a parent seemed a crucial factor in development of antisocial activity for some of those adolescents. The incidence of parental psychopathology was also higher than among other subjects of this study, and 30% of the natural fathers were alcoholic.

Despite the disrupted family background and interpersonal conflicts in the homes, the 20 adolescents' current functional parents (of whom there were 37), were generally people who cared about their children and had repeatedly sought help for them in appropriate ways.

Our study subjects were characterized by childhood restlessness, aggressivity, and scholastic underachievement. In late childhood and early adolescence they became precociously involved in smoking, drinking, sexual activity, driving cars, and rebelling against parental and scholastic restraints. The average age of onset of disruptive antisocial behavior was 12½ years, and the first hospital admission typically occurred three and one-half years later.

The clinical picture was dominated by school problems starting at an early age and continuing into high school with academic failure, fighting, truancy, and expulsion, usually occurring in that order. Arguments, alcohol use, temper tantrums, stealing, lying, running away, and vandalism led to serious conflicts with families and police. Disorders of mood or thought were not a prominent part of the clinical picture. Although nervousness, restlessness, and impatience were common complaints, depression and anxiety were typically related to frustrating or threatening circumstances which the patients' own behavior had brought about.

Hospitalization of the sociopathic psychiatric inpatients was usually occasioned by the immediate need for restraint of impulsive behavior or treatment of an acute toxic state. Hospitalization of the sociopathic adolescent controls on non-psychiatric wards was usually the result of traumatic injury suffered as the direct consequence of antisocial activity.

The patients were not hospitalized to provide definitive treatment of the long-standing personality disorder, but to alleviate the immediate problems which had precipitated admission. In addition, some of the patients, families, and physicians hoped that short-term psychiatric hospitalization and intensive evaluation would provide new therapeutic directions that could be pursued in other settings, for example, at home or in new schools or residential treatment centers.

REFERENCES

1. *DSM II: Diagnostic and Statistical Manual of Mental Disorders* (second edition). Washington, American Psychiatric Association 1968.
2. Robins, L. N. *Deviant Children Grown Up: A Sociological and Psychiatric Study of Antisocial Personality*. Baltimore, Williams and Wilkins Co., 1966.
3. Glueck, S., and Glueck, E. *Delinquents and Nondelinquents in Perspective*. Cambridge, Harvard University Press, 1968.
4. Perley, M., and Guze, S. B. Hysteria—the stability and usefulness of clinical criteria. N. Engl. J. Med. *266:* 421–426, 1962.
5. Guze, S. B., Wolfgram, E. D., McKinney, J. K., AND CANTWELL, D. P. Psychiatric illness in the families of convicted criminals. Dis. Nerv. Syst. *28:* 651–659, 1967.
6. Guze, S. B., Woodruff, R. A., and Clayton, P. J. Hysteria and antisocial behavior: further evidence of an association. Am. J. Psychiatry *127:* 957–960, 1971.
7. Cadoret, R. J. In *Textbook of Psychiatry* of ROCOM (subsidiary of Hoffmann-LaRoche, Inc.), Paul Miller, Ed. In press.
8. Robins, L. N. Social correlates of antisocial personality. Presented at the annual meeting of the American Sociological Association, New Orleans, August, 1972.
9. Dohrenwend, B. P., and Dohrenwend, B. S. *Social Status and Psychological Disorder: A Causal Inquiry*. New York, John Wiley and Sons, Inc., 1969.
10. McCord, W. and McCord, J. *The Psychopath*. New York, Van Nostrand Co., 1964.
11. Schulsinger, F. Psychopathy: heredity and environment. Int. J. Ment. Health. *1:* 190–206, 1972.
12. Morrison, J. R., and Stewart, M. A. A family study of the hyperactive child syndrome. Biol. Psychiatry *3:* 189–195, 1971.
13. Mendelson, W., Johnson, N., and Stewart, M. A. Hyperactive children as teenagers. J. Nerv. Ment. Dis. *153:* 273–279, 1971.
14. Liss, J. L., Welner, A., and Robins, E. Personality disorder: Part I. Record study. Br. J. Psychiatry *123:* 685–692, 1973.
15. Welner, A., Liss, J. L., and Robins, E. Personality disorder: Part II. Follow-up. Br. J. Psychiatry *124:* 359–366, 1974.

8

The "undiagnosed, unclassified" patient

CLASSIFICATION OF UNDIAGNOSED PATIENTS

As stated in Chapter 2, patients were called "undiagnosed" if they did not fit our strict criteria for classification according to syndromes which had been well established in the literature by systematic longitudinal and family studies. Sixty-two of the 110 psychiatric inpatients and 19 of the 110 controls were so designated, a total of 81 subjects. However, 50 of the 81 undiagnosed patients were subclassified according to the syndromes they most resembled, for example, "undiagnosed, most like depression," etc. Those 50 patients had failed to fulfill the diagnostic criteria for the syndromes only because of a paucity of symptoms or because of moderately atypical features which were not so striking as to make another diagnostic classification likely. The special term, "undiagnosed, schizoaffective," was used to designate seven acutely ill patients who had prominent features of both affective disorder and schizophrenia, so that neither diagnosis could be excluded. The undiagnosed patients who were classified according to the syndromes they most resembled have been discussed in chapters dealing with those syndromes.

After subclassification of the undiagnosed patients was completed, there remained 31 (29 psychiatric inpatients and two controls) who could not be so classified. There were 18 girls and 13 boys. In general, these 31 patients each had symptoms of more than one psychiatric syndrome, but in no case were symptoms of any one syndrome so dominant as to warrant classification according to that diagnosis. "Atypical" was an adjective often appearing in these patients' records. Their outcome at follow-up in adulthood should be of the greatest interest. In some cases, atypical precursors of typical syndromes may be identified. In other cases, new syndromes, for example, a personality disorder heretofore poorly described in the literature, may be delineated and found to have a consistent clinical course over time. Moreover, at follow-up the relative prognostic importance of different symptoms in adolescence may be clarified in a sample like this with a mixed clinical picture. For example, in patients who had both disturbed affect and delinquent behavior in their teens, we will be able to see whether one or both of these features remains predominant in adulthood, or whether the relative importance of one type of symptom diminishes with maturity. We will also be able to see whether new symptoms, for example, alcohol abuse in adulthood, are predictable on the basis of the clinical picture in adolescence. The results at follow-up may serve as a guide to more understanding and possibly more effective treatment of teenagers who do not conveniently fit into a diagnostic category and thus suffer from disorders whose outcome is not yet predictable.

GENERAL CONSIDERATIONS OF THE CLINICAL PICTURES AND BACKGROUNDS OF THE "UNDIAGNOSED, UNCLASSIFIED" GROUP

Since the "undiagnosed, unclassified" adolescents were a heterogeneous group, each case must be examined individually in order for the reader to get a true picture of the sample. This will be done later in this chapter. Nevertheless, a preliminary consideration of the group as a whole may be useful in giving the reader an idea of the constellation of symptoms affecting these patients and of the predominant problems in their social and family backgrounds. A "modal" undiagnosed, unclassified patient had a predominance of affective symptoms, but had an admixture of such behavioral problems as immaturity, argumentativeness, and rebelliousness. The group also had an earlier mean onset of illness (13.3 years, age at time of study 16.0 years) than patients with definite depression. In this respect they resembled the patients with antisocial personality more than they resembled patients with affective disorder. Illicit drug use played a definite or suspected role in the presenting picture of eight patients (26%), and may have contributed to the atypicality of the clinical course in those subjects. Moreover, most of the undiagnosed patients had a chaotic family background. This is similar to findings in patients with antisocial personality and hysteria.

Table 35 lists all psychiatric symptoms appearing in the present illnesses of more than a fourth of the undiagnosed, unclassified patients. The eight leading symptoms were those found among the leading symptoms of our typical depressives. Symptoms of argumentativeness and of academic and behavioral problems in school appear further down the list, with lesser frequency than among sociopaths, but with greater frequency than among the depressives, manics, and schizophrenics in our study. Auditory and visual hallucinations, reported by a significant minority of the undiagnosed, unclassified adolescents, did not have the vivid and persistent quality of hallucinations in schizophrenics. Rather, in some patients, they were evanescent, and in some patients we suspected that they were associated with drug use. In other patients, the reports of hallucinations

TABLE 35
Common Symptoms in Patients Who Were "Undiagnosed, Unclassified"
N = 31

Symptom	%
Depressed	65
Thoughts of suicide	65
Insomnia	61
Hopeless feelings	61
Crying	52
Suicide attempt, ever	48
Nervousness	45
Loss of appetite	45
Dizziness	39
Headaches	39
Arguing	39
Guilt feelings	39
Decreased interest	39
Worry	35
Held back in school	32
Auditory hallucinations	32
Trouble thinking or concentrating	32
Visual hallucinations	29
Truancy	29
Decreased ability in work or school	29
Expelled from school	26
Tired, weak	26
Running away from home overnight	26
Felt self to be a burden	26

seemed inconsistent with other aspects of the clinical picture, as if the patients were exaggerating the degree of their psychopathology.

We compared our undiagnosed, unclassified sample to the other patients in the study with respect to a number of items, for example, sex, race, and medical, social, and scholastic backgrounds. As a group they had a slightly, but not significantly, higher incidence of psychiatric disorders in their parents, and they had more scholastic and behavioral problems than other patients (except for sociopaths). When compared with the total study sample they were of equal intelligence (mean I.Q. = 110) but of somewhat lower socioeconomic status, although they were of higher social status than the adolescents with antisocial personality. None of these differences were striking, however. Rather the distinctive factor in the backgrounds of the undiagnosed, unclassified patients was the high incidence of chaos in their homes.

In only 17 cases, 55%, were both natural parents currently functioning in a parental role. In 12 cases (39%), the homes had either been broken by divorce (nine cases) or the patient placed for adoption (three cases). In two cases, when the mothers subsequently remarried they later separated from the patients' stepfathers. One natural father, one adoptive father, and one stepfather had died in the patients' lifetimes, and one natural father had been killed in the Korean War before the patient was born. The stepfather had been killed by the patient herself, a 15-year-old girl who had suffered much abuse at his hands over the years. In another case, the patient, also a 15-year-old girl, had shot her father in an unprovoked homicide attempt, totally blinding him. It is of interest that four deaths of parents or stepparents occurred in the cases of the 31 undiagnosed, unclassified, patients and six among the parents of the 20 sociopaths. Thus there were ten parental deaths for these 51 patients (20%) and only 11 for the other 169 subjects in our study (7%), $p < 0.05$.

One-third of the natural parents of undiagnosed, unclassified patients had had psychiatric illness. There were eight fathers and one mother who were alcoholic, two fathers with antisocial personality, five mothers with depression, and one father and four mothers with an undiagnosed psychiatric disorder. In addition, one stepfather drank heavily and another was quite abusive. The 21 ill natural parents were distributed among 16 families, so 52% of the 31 undiagnosed adolescents had at least one psychiatrically ill biologic parent. An additional patient had two brothers with antisocial personality and one with depression. Three patients had remote relatives who had committed suicide, but no first degree relatives had done so.

In all, 71% of the undiagnosed, unclassified patients had experienced major disruption in their relationship with parents either because of parental psychiatric illness, separation, divorce, desertion, death, or a combination of these factors. It would not be far-fetched to conclude that the great amount of psychiatric and social disruption in the immediate families of these patients played a role in the genesis or form of expression of the adolescents' psychiatric disorders. No other group in our study sample had such psychosocially chaotic backgrounds.

CONSIDERATION OF INDIVIDUAL CASES

Because of the clinical heterogeneity of the undiagnosed sample, meaningful generalizations cannot be made about the course of the illnesses, response to treatment, and so forth. Important information about all the undiagnosed, unclassified, patients is given in Table 36. We were unable to demonstrate correlations among age of onset, preexisting organic brain dysfunction, psychosocial disruption in the immediate family, and subsequent clinical picture. Not unexpectedly, suicide attempts were more frequent among the girls (12, 66%), than among the boys (three, 23%). By contrast, definite or suspected contribution of drugs to the clinical picture was present in six boys (46%) and only two girls (11%). The ages of onset of the undiagnosed disorders were difficult to ascertain for those patients in whom disturbances of behavior or mood began insidiously or several years in the past.

Representative case reports will aid readers in understanding this group.

The first patient had characteristics of both antisocial personality and depression.

Y-001—This 17-year-old white girl entered the hospital after a suicide attempt, having ingested barbiturates and aspirin. She had been self assertive, independent and tomboyish as a preschool child. When she was 11 years old her mother was hospitalized for depression, given ECT, and recovered. Marital troubles between the parents, present at least since the child was seven years old, worsened then. Her father, a certified public accountant, became irritable and drank excessively from the time the patient was 13 until she was 16. (The patient had several alcoholic relatives on the paternal side and a maternal great uncle, not an alcoholic, had hanged himself.)

By the time the patient was 13 years old she had begun to have conflicts with her parents over her desire for decreased restrictions on use of the telephone and on her freedom to go out. Her first suicide attempt (with 20 aspirin tablets) occurred after an argument with her father when she was 13. She told no one about this until a year later. During the subsequent four years the conflicts with her parents continued. Although she was bright (I.Q. 119), her school grades were below average. She began to steal items from stores regularly by age 14 and continued this practice until the time of admission.

At age 15, about a year and a half before admission, she began to have increasing nervousness, insomnia, impatience, and inability to keep still. By nine months before admission, age 17, she began to drink up to a fifth of whisky a week. She only became drunk once, however. Lying to her parents about her whereabouts became routine. Three or four months before admission, she began to have intercourse with her boyfriend, using no contraception because she wanted to become pregnant and "get away from home." In the few months before admission she ran away from home on two occasions and was brought back by the police. She became increasingly moody and lost weight. On the night before her admission she had an argument with her father, who took away her car keys. She felt hopeless, decided that life had no point if all she could do was "to sit and look at four walls like an old woman." She took 20 one-grain

Table 36

The "Undiagnosed, Unclassified" Patients

Patient	Sex	Race	Current Age	Coexisting Disorders	Probable Age Onset of Undiagnosed Disorder	Probable Duration of Undiagnosed Disorder	Disorders in Immediate Family	Clinical Features	Suicide Attempt?	Illicit Drugs' Contribution to Clinical Picture	Diagnoses Considered
Y-001	F	W	17	None	13	4 years	Mother had ECT for depression; father alcoholic. Parents had contemplated divorce	Depression, rebelliousness against parents	Yes		Depression; antisocial personality
Y-004	F	B	17	Mental deficiency, epilepsy	17	1 month	Natural mother unmarried. Patient adopted. Adoptive father died when patient 15	Recent frantic crying spells and multiple somatic complaints after stress			Hysteria; situational reaction
Y-006	F	W	18		18	2 months	Father alcoholic, deserted family; mother remarried	Devious; recent acute onset of tantrums after stress	Yes		Antisocial personality; situational reaction
Y-007	M	B	16		16	3 months		Irritability; sudden onset of transient muteness under stress			Depression; situational reaction
Y-008	F	W	15		15	Several months		Deviousness; shot father; reported hearing "voices"			Antisocial personality; schizophrenia
Y-011	M	W	16	Knocked out prior to onset	16	5 months		Headaches, irritability, poor concentration			Depression; brain concussion
Y-022	F	W	15		12	3 years	Natural father killed in war. Stepfather drank heavily. Brother hyperkinetic	Unhappy, irritable, school problems, suicide threats, "voices"	Yes		Hysteria; depression
Y-027	F	W	18		17	1½ to 2 years	Father alcoholic; sister hysteric	Demanding, manipulative, moody, temper outbursts, multiple somatic symptoms		(Alcohol)	Hysteria; depression
Y-028	F	W	13		12	9 months	Father alcoholic, beat wife, divorced	Manipulative suicide threats, deviousness, panicky spells	Yes		Epilepsy; antisocial personality; hysteria
Y-033	F	B	14	Epilepsy, organic brain syndrome	5	9 years	Father alcoholic, died of esophageal varices. Mother undiagnosed psychiatric disorder	Behavior problems for years	Yes		Depression

Y-034	F	W	19		14	5 years	Deserted by natural parents, age 13 months. Patient adopted	Sexual promiscuity, suicide threats, recent bizarre behavior		Probably	Antisocial personality; drug intoxication
Y-042	F	W	15		15	2 months	Natural parents divorced. Mother remarried. Patient killed abusive stepfather	Killed abusive stepfather. Some depressive symptoms			Depression
Y-044	F	W	18		17	1 year	Mother chronically nervous, poor health	Devious, defiant, depressed	Yes		Depression; antisocial personality
Y-050	M	W	17		16	15 months		Antisocial behavior; recent delusions	Yes	Probably	Depression; drug intoxication; schizophrenia
Y-051	F	W	12		6	6 years		School refusal with anxiety and nausea			Anxiety reaction
Y-053	M	W	14		10	4½ years	Mother chronically nervous	Depression, homosexuality, guarded			Depression
Y-057	M	W	17		15	2 years	Mother had ECT for depression	Behavior disorder, drug use, homosexuality	Yes	Yes	Antisocial personality; drug intoxication; depression
Y-061	M	W	15		14	14 months	One brother with depression, two with antisocial personality	Mixed affective symptoms, amphetamines	Yes	Yes	Manic-depressive disease; drug intoxication
Y-068	F	B	19		16	3 years	Natural parents divorced; natural mother subsequently separated from stepfather	Deviousness, distraught, somatic complaints, "seeing and hearing things"	Yes	Probably	Hysteria; depression; drug intoxication
Y-075	F	W	17		15	2 years	Mother had depression; father alcoholic. Parents divorced. Mother remarried	Temper tantrums, depression, hostile to parents	Yes		Depression; hysteria
Y-083	M	W	16		16	10 months	Father alcoholic. Parents divorced. Mother remarried, then separated	Running away, amnesia			Antisocial personality
Y-085	F	W	15		7	8 years	Natural parents both alcoholic; patient adopted age 7	Antisocial behavior, intercourse with adoptive father, "voices"	Yes		Antisocial personality; schizophrenia
Y-095	F	W	15	Nephrotic syndrome, steroids	12	3 years	Father antisocial personality. Shot at mother. Mother "nervous." Parents divorced	Depression, manipulative, hostile, many somatic symptoms	Yes		Depression; hysteria; antisocial personality
Y-097	M	W	18		17	8 months	Mother depressed	Depression, hostility to family		Probably	Depression; drug intoxication
Y-100	M	W	19		15	4 years		Depression, drugs		Yes	Depression; drug intoxication
Y-102	M	B	13	Hyperkinetic since age 3	11	2 years	Parents separated for past 5 years. Mother, anxiety and depression	Hyperkinetic, antisocial aggressiveness. Bizarre spells, ? glue sniffing		Probably	Antisocial personality; drug intoxication

TABLE 36—*Continued*

Patient	Sex	Race	Current Age	Coexisting Disorders	Probable Age Onset of Undiagnosed Disorder	Probable Duration of Undiagnosed Disorder	Disorders in Immediate Family	Clinical Features	Suicide Attempt?	Illicit Drugs' Contribution to Clinical Picture	Diagnoses Considered
Y-106	F	W	17	Mental deficiency	16	4 months	Father antisocial. Parents divorced. Brother mentally defective. Patient raised by various relatives. Other siblings given up for adoption	Temper outbursts, suicidal threats, slowed behavior	Yes		Depression; epilepsy
Y-107	F	W	18		13	5 years		Former depression, recent increase in energy, ? delusions of reference	Yes		Manic-depressive disease; hysteria; schizophrenia
Y-110	M	W	15	Bitten by hog prior to onset	14	15 months		Depression, auditory hallucinations, "passivity feelings," dizzy, falling			Organic brain syndrome; schizophrenia
C-006	M	B	12		12	1 month		Anxiety, irritability, insomnia			Depression; anxiety neurosis
C-077	M	W	16	Massive obesity (325 pounds)	8	8 years	Father nervous, easily upset	School underachievement, few friends. Demanding personality, headaches			"Personality disorder"

Butisol tablets and six aspirin at 11:00 p.m. She was difficult to arouse at 8:00 a.m. when her father awakened her. She then told him of the suicide attempt and was admitted to the hospital.

Moderately depressed upon admission, she improved on psychotherapy during her 25 day hospitalization. In outpatient treatment over the next few months her situation fluctuated, with rebellious behavior coinciding with her father's pressure upon her, and apparently stimulated by it. By nine months after discharge the home situation was more peaceful and she had markedly improved.

The next patient had preexisting brain damage and a bizarre response to emotional stress which led to hospitalization at age 17.

Y-004—This 17-year-old black girl was born prematurely, the third child of an unmarried 15-year-old girl, and adopted at three weeks of age. When she was four to six weeks old she had a series of four or five convulsions. She walked at one year of age, began to speak at two years, but was noted to be mentally defective when she entered primary school. Thereafter she remained in special schools, where she had chronic mild disciplinary problems.

At age 13, following a fall in which she struck her head, she began to have spells of shaking and twitching without loss of consciousness. An electroencephalogram showed paroxysmal activity. She was placed on anticonvulsant medications, and the spells stopped.

When she was 15, her adoptive father died. She experienced much fright at seeing him in the coffin, fearing he would "rise up." At times over the next two years she would "see him standing by the bed at night and hear him mumbling."

At age 17, five weeks before admission, a new school year began. She proved unable to learn what was being taught in the special school and became a serious behavior problem, throwing things and beating up other children. (She was quite large for her age.) This led to her expulsion. "When school began this year, I couldn't go because they said I was too stupid. When I was at school, I couldn't learn fast enough, they said. I was scared of everybody. They made fun of me." She abruptly developed insomnia and pains in her flank, back, and abdomen, radiating into her vagina. "I think I'm losing weight. I'm very nervous. All this is a lot worse at night. When I hurt at night, I want to die." She cried, shook, and took to bed during the month prior to admission. Medical workups in the clinic were negative. Finally, increased shaking, combativeness, and vomiting led to her admission to Renard Hospital.

Upon admission she was overactive, cried, attempted to run away, and grimaced frequently. Her right arm and hand shook rhythmically four times per second. All the abnormal movements and distraught affect stopped whenever the patient was temporarily distracted or reassured, only to begin again upon slight provocation or frustration. Defective intelligence was obvious in conversation, and she had a childish manner, even when calm.

During a 13-day hospitalization the patient became calmer and cheerful. She was treated with chlordiazapoxide and diphenylhydantoin, and provisions for further education were made.

The following patient had clinical traits suggesting both antisocial personality and schizophrenia.

Y-008—This 15-year-old white girl was admitted to Renard Hospital because she had shot her father, blinding him.

She was the youngest of five children of a family in a rural community. Her medical history was unremarkable except for brief periods of delirium with fever at age 11 and 14. When the patient was about 12 she began to be devious concerning the breaking of restrictions against seeing boys. This continued over the next three years.

Both the family and the patient stated that she had reported dreams of seeing her uncle in a coffin on the night before he died, when the patient was eight years old, and a similar dream before her grandmother's death when the patient was 15. She stated that five months before admission she heard the voices of her uncle and grandmother telling her not to worry, "the family would be together soon." This frightened her, but she came to believe it was not a strange occurrence. Aside from recurrent dreams of her grandfather killing her grandmother, she reported no other bizarre mental phenomena until just prior to admission.

By age 15, a few months before admission, she had begun to have conflicts with her parents concerning a "wild" boyfriend. On one occasion she even ran away from home briefly to be with him, but rejoined her family instead of meeting him. An intimate correspondence between the patient and boyfriend was found by the parents and disturbed them greatly. One letter from him said "we can get married when those two obstacles are removed." It was not specified what, or who, the objects were. However, she seemed more content in the three months prior to admission, improved in her schoolwork, and got along better with her parents.

One week before she shot her father she began to have dreams about seeing him in a coffin, which frightened her. Four days before the shooting, she called her parents to her bed at night, clung to them and cried out, over and over, "Don't let Daddy die!" On the night of the shooting the patient stated that she went to her father who was watching television and asked him "Do you want a sody?" (soda) He did not reply, but continued to watch television, ignoring her. She repeated the question over and over, but he just continued to laugh at the television program. She became very angry. "He never even knew I was around. He never paid attention to any of us. Always complaining about how much trouble we were. Then a roaring noise filled all the rooms of the house. The good Lord put it there to make people slow down. Everybody was going too fast." She heard God's voice like an echo, saying "______, you've got to do something." The roaring noise was terrible, threatening to smother her, and she said she had to do something to make it stop. She got a .22 rifle, came up beside her father and pointed it at him, thinking "I can't do it. I'll miss him a mile." Then he turned slightly, and she thought he saw her. At that moment, since there was no way for her to explain why she was standing there with a gun, she decided to kill him, and pulled the trigger.

The bullet severed both optic nerves. He jumped from his seat unaware of what had happened, as he had not really seen his daughter with the gun, and called out to his wife "I can't see!" The daughter had left the room and put away the gun by the time her mother entered. The father was standing by his chair with blood all over his face. During that night the patient was upset and crying, but she did not admit to the shooting until questioned by the police some days later. They had previously suspected an unknown intruder of the assault but soon concluded that the shot must have been fired by the wife or the daughter, and they finally elicited an admission from the latter.

Upon entering the hospital, the patient had a bland affect, admitting to only a hazy memory of the shooting. She gave the above detailed account after an intravenous injection of amytal. During that interview she showed much emotion and spoke of loving and hating her father. She said that killing him "might help God because Daddy never goes to church," and that if he were out of the way, her mother might more readily understand her feelings for her boyfriend. She expressed remorse, stating that she would need to talk with God about what she should do to atone for hurting her father, an act that had been inspired "by the Devil . . . maybe I'll work hard or something to make up for it."

During hospitalization she showed generally bland affect, no signs of depression, thought disorder, or hallucinations. She met with her family, who preferred to believe (despite her confession) that not she, but an intruder, had fired the shot. She seemed devious and associated with teenagers on the ward who had antisocial behavior problems. She was transferred from Renard Hospital to the St. Louis State Hospital's adolescent unit, where she entered training as a cosmetician and beautician in the vocational program as a day patient. She was consistently hostile toward her parents. She eloped from the State Hospital's jurisdiction nine months after the shooting and disappeared.

The next patient had symptoms of a behavior disorder and depression, as well as bizarre features raising the suspicion that she might have early schizophrenia.

Y-022—This white girl was 15 when she was admitted to Renard Hospital after a suicide attempt.

Her father had been killed in the Korean War before she was born. Her mother had remarried when the patient was one year old. The stepfather had some intermittent heaving drinking. During her childhood the patient was "never happy." She cried a great deal and habitually vomited in the morning before going to school. Conflicts with her father were the rule.

The patient stated that beginning in early childhood she had heard strange, foreign voices talking to her, sometimes accompanied by visions of faces. She said that the voices, which she did not characterize as having the quality of true, audible voices, sometimes caused her to scream when she was a young child. But by her mid-teens these phenomena had become less and less frequent, finally stopping (until just before her admission to Renard Hospital). She said she had thought little about the voices as a child, accepting them as a common feature of her life.

At age 12, she began to exhibit troublesome behavior, becoming noisy, having temper tantrums, and doing poorly in school. She would scream at strangers, using foul language. On occasions she threw eggs at people. She was at times truant from school. Concomitantly, she seemed depressed, and by age 12 she began to express suicidal thoughts. She began weekly psychotherapy then, but neither that nor changes of schools seemed to help her mood or behavior. By age 14, she had become more socially withdrawn. She developed insomnia and increasingly persistent suicidal thoughts during that year before admission. "Life is crappy, boring; people are uninteresting." She gradually lost interest in things. Four months before admission she tried to take a handful of aspirin after an argument with her father, but was prevented from doing so. Three weeks before admission she took 18 aspirin without telling anyone. Finally, on the day before admission she was found by her mother, making tentative slashes on her wrists with a razor blade. She was hospitalized because of this. In general, over the years her stormy responses to situations seemed strange and out of proportion to the degree of provocation. There was no history of drug use.

Upon admission she was moody, at times truculent, at times giggling. She said that she hoped to kill herself. There was a discrepancy between her statements about her affective distress and the apparent shallowness of her outward expression of emotion. During hospitalization she continued to have suicidal preoccupation and inappropriate affect, and said that she heard voices. She did not improve significantly during a five-week stay and was readmitted with the same symptoms one month after discharge. During that admission she improved on chlorpromazine.

In the patient described below, a clinical picture initially resembling sociopathy was altered by the abuse of drugs. The extent of this abuse was unknown to the parents. In fact, heavy use was denied by the patient himself, yet we had a strong suspicion that drugs were responsible for the more bizzare symptoms. The case demonstrated how toxic effect of drugs might lead the psychiatrist astray in his diagnosis and treatment if, as is often true, the patient is not frank in giving a history of drug abuse.

Y-050—This 17-year-old white boy was the son of a psychologist in in the Armed Forces. There was no family history of psychiatric illness or marital disruption. His parents described him as having been a warm, happy child who was non-conformist and who underachieved in school. Unknown to them, he stole many items from stores in his early teens, selling some of them. He lied frequently and cheated regularly in school. Once, when he was 14, he ran away overnight after conflict with his parents. By age 15, he was progressively losing interest in school and began to fail subjects.

Both the patient and his parents said that a definite change occurred when he was 16, from 12 to 17 months before admission. However, the parents and the boy gave different versions of the history. The mother and father noticed primarily a change in the direction of social deviance, "a breakdown of character." He began to tell more obvious lies, was non-communicative, lost his former interest in wildlife and became interested in the guitar. He let his hair grow long and neglected personal hygiene. He slept excessively, was guarded and defensive, and over the year prior to admission became openly defiant of restrictions on his activities. Four days before admission he left school, saying he felt "closed in." Two days before admission he ran away from home, leaving behind a note saying he was going to Boston to see the World's Series (although he had no interest in baseball). His parents had him picked up by police in Illinois, and he was admitted to the Renard Hospital.

The patient's story was different in quality, although he also dated the change as beginning about one year before admission. He stated that a conflict with his father over curfew hours altered his attitude at that time. He began to worry more than usual, resented his parents, and lost interest in his former pursuits. By six months before admission, he was having trouble concentrating on his schoolwork, seeing little importance to it. At that time too, around his 17th birthday, he developed insomnia and a fear of thinking personal thoughts when others were in the room. He could "hear" his own thoughts at times arguing with him in his head. Over the next six months prior to admission he said he began to use drugs—bromides, mescaline, marijuana, benzedrine, and cough syrup containing antihistamines—but in telling his history he minimized the extent of their use. His symptoms and his manner of telling the history suggested that he was withholding information about the extent of his drug abuse.

About four months before admission he had visual illusions at night on one occasion, his arms felt like rubber, and he heard a voice saying "This is what we're going to do." After that he developed a feeling of being followed and plotted against. At about that time, he was elated for two or three days after a dose of mescaline and decided to tell people about the effects of psychedelic drugs so that they could experience their "mind-expanding" properties. Subsequently, he began to interpret words of popular songs on the radio as having special significance for him. At times he believed they were messages from God.

Two months before admission he began to want to die. At the same time he developed a sense of unreality and the paradoxic feeling of deriving great appreciation from little things. As the school year started, one month before admission, he began to have disciplinary problems at school for episodes of misbehavior. Resentfulness against peers and parents increased and he began to fear that his father would kill him. At that time, he also experienced episodes of pleasant visual imagery when he closed his eyes. He felt himself to be in a trance. During the few days before he left for Boston "to see the World's Series," he admitted to taking several sleeping pills (in a suicide attempt), two bottles of cough syrup at one time, and getting intoxicated by the use of an inhaler containing benzedrine. Suicide thoughts were prominent during those days, he said, but the interviewer doubted their seriousness.

In the hospital he was polite and cooperative at first. There was no evidence for marked affective disturbance. He continually pushed for greater hospital privileges, threatened to elope from the ward on one occasion, and questioned the nurses about whether he would get "high" if he took 10 imipramine tablets. He had not changed significantly by the time of discharge to outpatient therapy. At no time in the hospital did he exhibit symptoms suggestive of schizophrenia.

The following patient also had a history of drug (amphetamine) use, but only for a brief period earlier in his illness. His case was somewhat suggestive of manic-depressive disorder but there were too many atypical features to classify him diagnostically.

Y-061—This white boy was 15 when admitted to Renard Hospital for depressive symptoms. He had a family history of psychiatric disorder—one brother who had probable depression, two with antisocial personality, a maternal great grandmother who had multiple state hospital admissions, and a maternal cousin who had committed suicide by shooting himself when he was an adolescent.

The patient's premorbid personality was described by himself as friendly, but with few close companions. His mother described him as "always uncoordinated" physically, and as a loner with only one friend and no special interests, either in school or out.

At the age of 13, two years before admission, he began to make up stories about things he had done, in order to brag. His parents noticed a quality of stubbornness beginning at about that time. Later in that school year (eighth grade), he began to refuse to go to gym class at school and used devious means to avoid it. At that time he was accused by his school principal of using drugs, but denied it. There was no evidence for it at the time.

In the subsequent summer, as he turned 14, he developed a period of elation, which lasted a couple of months. During this time he organized an Optimist Club branch for boys and got by with only four hours sleep at night. This phase was succeeded by a three-month period of withdrawal, decreased communication with his parents, fatiguability, disagreements with teachers, and some truancy. This depression began about one year prior to the Renard Hospital admission. He made a suicide attempt with 24 over-the-counter sleeping pills early in the course of the depression, but told no one of this at the time. He also began masturbation fairly openly at home. If anyone was in the room, he would simply throw a sheet over himself. He went into the bathroom on numerous occasions and would emerge "completely out of breath." Toward the end of this three-month period of depression he bought "pep pills" of unknown strength through illegal channels and began to feel better after taking about nine pills per day for perhaps one week. He denied subsequent illegal drug use, but there is, of course, the possibility that some drugs were used again during the several months before admission. His depression had lifted, although the open masturbation continued during the year prior to admission, and he evaded his father's attempts to discuss it with him.

There ensued a period of relative well being, lasting approximately four months. But, toward the end of that school year (9th grade), he once more lost interest in school, developed antagonism to his teachers, truanted 10 or 12 times, and failed courses. At that time he was worrying a great deal about his brother, who had been wounded in Viet Nam.

During the ensuing summer vacation he felt better, but as the new school year approached, one month before admission, he developed apprehension about returning to classes. He became depressed, irritable, tired, sleepless, and lost weight. He dropped out of school two days after beginning the 10th grade, but continued his job selling magazines and sought psychiatric help at the Washington University Clinic without telling his parents. The psychiatrist contacted the parents, and the patient entered treatment, receiving antidepressants as an outpatient for three weeks without improvement. His agitation and insomnia continued, and he began to speak of death as inevitable, something he might as well get over with. As a result, he was admitted to the hospital.

Upon admission he was depressed and irritable with little spontaneous speech. There was no evidence of hallucinations or delusions, but suicidal ideation was prominent. He was relatively uncommunicative about his depressed feelings, which often had to be inferred from his withdrawn behavior and references to death. His physician was most impressed with the symptoms suggesting affective disorder, despite the history of behavior problems, the admitted abuse of drugs (at least on an earlier occasion), and despite one childish-appearing attempt to elope from the hospital. Therefore, he was given a course of electrotherapy. He showed marked improvement and was discharged after a stay of 51 days.

SUMMARY

The "Undiagnosed, Unclassified" Patient

Thirty-one adolescents (29 psychiatric inpatients and two controls) could not be classified according to established psychiatric syndromes. Each had symptoms of two or more syndromes or atypical features which made classification impossible. Affective symptoms were most prominent in the group as a whole, and suicide attempts had occurred in 48%. Several had character traits of "immaturity," independent of their affective symptoms, and had a history of scholastic and behavior problems. Illicit drug use played a definite or suspected role in the clinical pictures of eight patients (26%) and may have contributed to the atypicality of the course of illness in those subjects. There was a striking amount of psychosocial instability in the immediate families of the adolescents who were "undiagnosed, unclassified." For example, in 52% one or both parents had had psychiatric disorders. A total of 71% had suffered major disruptions in the relationship with one or both parents: parental psychopathology, separation, divorce, desertion, or death, or a combination of these deprivation experiences.

However, these patients did not form a clinically homogeneous sample, and it would be misleading (or premature) to lend too much weight to general characteristics of the group. The individual features of each case are outlined in Table 36, and six cases are presented in more detailed reports. Follow-up information about the fate of these "undiagnosed, unclassified," subjects in adulthood, and their clinical and social histories in the intervening years, will be of great interest. Their outcome is less certain than that of any other group in our study, since they do not belong to a syndrome whose course is, within certain limits, predictable. Thus from the follow-up new information may be gained concerning the appropriate classification and treatment of youngsters with mixed and atypical symptom pictures.

9

Treatment of psychiatrically ill adolescents

INTRODUCTION

The investigation reported in this book was not a controlled study of treatment. Nevertheless, it is important to include a chapter about therapy, a subject of great interest to the author and many readers. The information and opinions in this chapter were derived from observations made by the author during the course of this study, as well as from experience with his own patients and from reading the works of other writers.

Of necessity this chapter will cover broad territory. Several syndromes and modes of therapy will be discussed. It would be insufficient to deal only with the treatment of those adolescents considered in our study, all of whom were inpatients. Most adolescents who need psychiatric treatment will never be inpatients, and the great majority of those who must at times be in hospitals are there only briefly before returning to homes, schools, jobs, and outpatient treatment.

Since most people who treat troubled adolescents are not psychiatrists, this chapter is not addressed exclusively to members of that specialty. The author hopes that others working in the field of treatment and counseling —non-psychiatric physicians, psychologists, social workers, clergymen, activity therapists, guidance counselors, juvenile officers, and teachers— may find this book useful in some respects. An attempt has been made to avoid the use of jargon peculiar to any specialty.

Many readers, whether in psychiatry or other fields, do not place as much emphasis as we do on the process of diagnosing patients according to specific syndromes. As discussed in Chapter 2, we did this whenever possible, because previous longitudinal clinical investigations and studies of patients' relatives have demonstrated that most psychiatrically ill patients can be classified according to well established diagnostic categories. Such classification provides important clues about proper treatment and probable outcome. In any case, a syndrome-oriented frame of reference, if used properly, does no violence to an adolescent's individuality. Use of a "medical model" does not prevent a social, psychodynamic, or family-oriented approach to the emotionally disturbed youngster. The author believes that all these factors must be given consideration, and that if a professional person works with teenagers inflexibly and ignores either diagnostic realities or intrapersonal and interpersonal dynamics, he may do more harm than good for the people he is trying to help.

GENERAL CONSIDERATIONS

Preparation of the Physician or Counselor

Making a diagnosis, whether of the teenager's psychiatric syndrome or of a noxious environmental situation, is of primary importance. Any professional who works with emotionally disturbed adolescents should be armed with the ability to do this. This requires that he be familiar with the natural histories of the different syndromes, know which questions to ask, and interview patients and relatives systematically. Diagnosing a psychiatric disorder is not a terribly difficult skill for an intelligent person to learn with instruction and experience. It does not require a medical education.

Second, the counselor or physician should be acquainted with resources for helping teenagers in his own community and with some of the educational and treatment resources in other parts of the country. He should develop mutually cooperative relationships with: hospitals, including those offering somatic therapies and short-term intervention and those providing residential treatment; outpatient facilities, both clinics and individual physicians or other therapists who work with adolescents; schools, public, private, and specialized; juvenile courts, and their counseling and educational systems and detention facilities; and organizations providing jobs and vocational training. Contact with various lay organizations, for example, youth crisis intervention services and drug counseling groups, may also be helpful. Of all these resources, liaison with medical facilities and schools are of primary importance. Unless the physician or counselor lives in a very large metropolitan areas, he will probably find that local facilities are inadequate to meet the needs of some of his patients. Contact with physicians and schools in other communities may be essential to the proper practice of adolescent psychiatry.

Third, the professional who works with troubled adolescents should be flexible, and he should possess common sense, the most essential ingredient of psychotherapy and the best safeguard against some of the foolish notions that at times prevail in the field of psychiatry.

Initial Evaluation of the Adolescent

The initial evaluation of the psychiatrically ill teenager is an intensive process, but one which can usually be completed in one or two days. Two comprehensive interviews, one with the patient himself and one (separately) with a knowledgeable informant, almost always provide sufficient information for an accurate understanding of the case, so long as the interviews are conducted properly and the patient and informant are not both deliberately distorting the history. New information will be forthcoming on subsequent interviews as the patient develops more rapport with his interviewer and as data arrive from such diverse sources as schools, probation officers, physicians, laboratories, and so forth. But it is the initial evaluation which provides the crucial information. In the author's experience, it is only rarely that the diagnosis and attendant life problems of an adolescent are not discovered or strongly suspected after the first systematic interviews of patient and informant are completed. A treatment plan can usually be instituted on the first day of contact between a teenager and the person who is trying to help him.

The author customarily interviews the teenager first, alone, regardless of how disturbed he may be. This should help demonstrate to the patient that the actions being taken are primarily on his behalf, whether he sought the consultation voluntarily or was brought there partly or totally against his will.

The accompanying parent or other informant may then be interviewed alone, with the interviewer respecting the patient's confidence except insofar as disclosure of confidential material might prevent death or serious injury. After interviewing the informant, the physician or other counselor should see the adolescent again either alone or with the informant, depending on the circumstances, to make recommendations and outline a plan of treatment.

The First Interview

This chapter will not provide details of the techniques and content of the diagnostic interview. A number of text books give such information, and the research interview from this study is provided in Appendix I. However, some general comments, which apply to the interviews of both patient and informants, are in order here.

The author has found it most helpful to orient the first part of the interview around the *specific events and symptoms* leading to the consultation, and the exact reasons why consultation was sought now, rather than at some other time. The initial phase of this discussion should be as open-ended as possible, so that the interview is elicited from the patient or informant, not imposed upon him. The person being interviewed is encouraged to give a spontaneous chronologic account of recent symptoms and life circumstances, with his account uncontaminated by the interviewer's preconceptions about what is wrong with him. This procedure has several advantages: first, responsibility for giving the history is assigned to the patient, and he is forced to think about what has happened to him and to try to make it make sense to an outside observer. Second, the patient's real priorities and goals, however unreasonable they may appear to the interviewer, can be learned early in the course of treatment, before they are influenced by the interviewer's expectations of the patient. Third, a spontaneous account early in the interview serves as an excellent opportunity for a mental status examination. The interviewer can observe thought processes, thought content, degree of orientation, general level of intelligence, behavioral abnormalities, affect, and so forth, as well as elicit information about key symptoms and life circumstances. Thus the early spontaneous part of the interview is a great time-saver, eliminating the need for many of the "check list" and standard mental status questions later in the interview. It would be absurd, for example, to ask a patient to interpret proverbs if he has, while giving a spontaneous and relevant history of the present illness, demonstrated above-average intelligence and a total absence of bizarre thought content.

Some adolescents are very reluctant to give a history. In such cases the interviewer may be tempted to begin, prematurely, a check list of questions which have "yes" or "no" as the answers. Such a procedure almost guarantees that the patient will not open up, and the interviewer may never hear the patient's own story. For these patients it is especially important that the interviewer hold out as long as possible for a spontaneous history and encourage, rather than stifle, the patient's responsibility for giving his own account. It is often helpful to begin the interview with such a reluctant talker by asking questions to which the patient must certainly know the answer. For example, an adolescent who replies "I don't know" when he is asked why he was brought to the therapist can hardly give the same response to the question "Who came with you?," unless he pleads loss of memory. By such devices a friendly interviewer may gradually induce the shy, suspicious, or resentful teenager to talk more and more openly about important aspects of his history. Of course, some patients will be so antagonistic or so seriously ill that the therapist will not obtain a reliable interview, despite his patience and persistence.

With other patients, the interviewer may encounter the opposite problem in the early, open-ended portion of the interview. The patient may be overly loquacious, rambling on in excessive detail. In those cases, the interviewer must intervene to help the patient stick to a relevant account of those recent symptoms and circumstances which the patient himself believes are of primary importance. It may require some skill on the part of the interviewer to keep from suppressing the patient's spontaneity while preventing time consuming and irrelevant circumlocution.

After the early, open-ended part of the interview, the interviewer should carefully follow up the leads presented by the patient in his spontaneous account. In this way, the therapist can round out his understanding of the present illness and relevant life circumstances. The interviewer must try to determine the chronology and consequences of every important symptom and event mentioned. Only in this way can he discover the answer to the question that is most crucial to choice of treatment and prediction of outcome in each case: *in what ways, and for how long, has the patient been different from his usual self?*

Following the completion of the accounts of present illness and current life circumstances, the interviewer will need to ask systematically a series of questions (varying according to what is wrong with the patient and what the patient has omitted from his spontaneous account) about psychiatric and medical symptoms and other items in the personal, social, family, and scholastic histories. When possible, it is best to ask such questions in a manner that encourages the patient to elaborate, rather than to answer with a "yes" or "no." To omit this systematic questioning is to do the patient a great disservice, as it may leave the physician in ignorance about matters of great importance. It is nonsense to assert, as some writers have done, that such interrogation impairs rapport and may obstruct the conduct of therapy. If the questioning is done in a sensitive manner with due respect for the patient's feelings, and if the importance of such questioning is explained, the process can contribute to rapport with the patient. It can demonstrate that the therapist takes him quite seriously as a person and is interested in many aspects of his life and feelings which have not formerly been inquired about. In the author's experience, the first or second interview is the ideal time for detailed inquiry. The opportunity to ask a broad series of questions may never again present itself, and the physician may ultimately fail to know his patient completely enough if he does not interview him quite systematically at the very beginning of their relationship.

Immediate Treatment Plans, with Special Reference to Hospitalization

Following the initial evaluation, the recommendations which the therapist makes to the patient and his family will obviously depend upon the diagnosis and the individual circumstances of the case. Treatment of patients with specific conditions will be discussed later, but something should be said here about the issue of hospitalization.

In some quarters, psychiatric hospitalization of adolescents has been denigrated as unnecessary or harmful, with the allegation that it is merely a means by which the doctor and the family avoid approaching the "real" problems of the patient, or that it fosters undue dependency in an artificial setting. To some extent, this view represents a healthy reaction to the practice of institutionalizing the children of wealthy families, simply for prolonged, expensive inpatient psychotherapy, or the practice or relegating extremely troublesome (perhaps psychotic or sociopathic) teenagers to the back wards of state hospitals where they may be lost among a herd of relatively neglected chronic patients. But it would be a great mistake to consider abandonment of the practice of hospitalization altogether, since it may at times be the only practical way of dealing with the real problem, and since it may prove life-saving and prevent severe disruption of the patient's family and serious complications of his illness.

In the author's view, hospitalization is indicated for protection of a patient's life or limb, when active treatment cannot be practically effected in an outpatient setting, and when the physician has clearly in mind the specific goals of hospitalization. Thus the psychiatrically ill adolescent should be admitted to a hospital: when suicide is a serious possibility; when the patient's behavior is disruptive and unmanageable by people outside the hospital; when, even in the absence of disruptive behavior, neither the patient nor his family have the capacity to cooperate in the current phase of treatment; or when a diagnostic workup, possibly requiring medical and neurologic as well as psychiatric investigation, can more safely and expeditiously be accomplished in a hospital setting. Judicious use of the psychiatric hospital can save lives, time, money, and trouble, and should be a resource which is directly or indirectly available to all professional persons working with troubled teenagers.

TREATMENT OF SPECIFIC CONDITIONS

Depression

Unless the depressed teenager is suicidal, or behaving with such poor judgment that his life is disrupted and his future well being compromised, or requires electroconvulsive therapy, he should usually be treated as an outpatient. This will prevent undue interruption of his schoolwork or home life. At times, of course, such an interruption may be indicated, when the environmental situation is clearly making matters worse for the patient.

Grief and Bereavement Reactions

Symptoms of depression may arise in formerly well persons who encounter objectively severe stress or loss—serious medical illness, rejection by a lover, death of a relative, etc. It is not yet clear whether this "depressive symptom complex" (as Clayton[1] calls it) is in some essential way the same thing as a severe depressive illness attended by such symptoms as vegetative changes, delusions of worthlessness, and illogical despair. Psychiatric care is sought by only a minority of those suffering such reactions of grief and distress,[1] which are probably common in the population.

However, psychiatrists and counselors are sometimes called upon to see previously stable adolescents with these reactions which may, especially in teenage girls, be accompanied by suicidal threats or attempts. Short-term psychotherapy is indicated for these youths. The therapist should be supportive while at the same time helping the patient explore the personal significance and consequences of the stressful event. In this way, the adolescent may be helped to resolve the grief and conflicts engendered by the situation and resume his social and scholastic productivity. Antidepressant drugs are seldom indicated for this condition, which is usually brief in duration and not attended by symptoms other than the mood disturbance itself. At most, the author occasionally uses mild tranquilizers, such as diazepam or chlordiazepoxide, when the reaction is accompanied by tension and insomnia. Pharmacologically very potent drugs such as tricyclic antidepressants or barbiturates may add nothing to such a patient except the experience of their side effects, and may occasionally prove dangerous if the patient impulsively decides to take an overdose.

Depressive Illness

Depressive illness, in which the changes in the patient include dysphoria (whose duration and severity may make no sense in terms of stress) as well as other mental and physiologic symptoms (Chapter 4), is another matter altogether. Supportive psychotherapy is always indicated, as well as reassurance that the condition will remit and is not the patient's fault. Deep and stressful exploration of psychologic conflicts should be deferred in adolescents who are temporarily suffering from illogical feelings of guilt and worthlessness. Suicidal potential must be ascertained (see below), and the initial phases of treatment should be carried out in the hospital if there is a risk that the patient might kill himself.

In such cases, it makes no sense to withhold tricyclic antidepressants, whose efficacy has been well demonstrated. If they are prescribed, they should not be given sporadically or in small doses, or they might as well not be given at all. Adolescents will require dosages as high as those given to adults, up to 300 mgm. of imipramine daily, for example (Klein and Davis[2]). Moreover, an adequate trial of a tricyclic antidepressant must consist of a high dose, given for a least three weeks, before the physician can justifiably conclude that he has tried the drug and that it has not worked. It must also be explained to the patient and his family that an antidepressant does not take effect after a single dose, and that uninterrupted use of the medicine for two or three weeks is necessary before therapeutic effects are experienced. Once the symptoms of depression have been alleviated, the effective dose should be maintained for a couple of months, then tapered off gradually. It is not unusual for an untreated episode of depressive illness to run a course of several months' duration before remitting spontaneously. Thus when symptoms have been pharmacologically suppressed by tricyclic drugs, they may be expected to return if the dose of antidepressant is reduced prematurely. The physician does not know in advance how long his patient's depression is going to last and should follow him closely as long as he requires any medication and as long as any symptoms endure.

The patient and his family should be cautioned against decisions involving significant life changes while the patient is seriously depressed and his judgment impaired. For example, it is not unusual for a depressed adolescent to conclude that the pressures of schoolwork caused his illness (even if academic pressures in his past were not attended by depression). He might be tempted to withdraw from school because of this, or change to an easier school or curriculum. But, while he is ill, he may be quite unable to assess the wisdom of such decisions, and regret them after his recovery.

The use of electroconvulsive therapy in depressive illness should be reserved for those patients who have failed to respond to an adequate trial on antidepressants; for those who are imminent suicidal risks even in the hospital, so that it is too dangerous to wait two or three weeks for antidepressants to take effect; for those whose symptoms include prominent delusions (since antidepressants are less often effective in patients with severely disordered content of thought); for those who are suffering such agony that it is unkind to wait for an antidepressant drug to work; and for those who have symptoms which might produce serious complications unless prompt intervention is begun by ECT. Such symptoms include, for example, stupor, extreme agitation with exhaustion, and refusal or inability to eat or drink.

If electroconvulsive therapy is to be given, eight to 12 treatments are usually necessary, and some patients require more. Marked improvement after the first few treatments, which is not uncommon, should not tempt the physician to discontinue this form of therapy after three of four treatments. In those cases, the patient will probably relapse, and the physician will need to begin the entire process over again. When a course of ECT is successfully completed, the doctor may need to devote even more attention to his patient for a time. Some depressive symptoms may remain, necessitating antidepressant drug therapy. In addition, the patient may suffer from temporary memory loss, confusion, and emotional lability as side effects of the convulsions. Proper treatment may include continued hospitalization for a week or more after the last ECT treatment, supportive psychotherapy, reassurance, explanations to the patient about what has happened to him, and protection of the patient from the consequences of poor judgment or premature resumption of school, job, and general social contacts. Close follow-up is necessary after a course of electrotherapy. The doctor is not doing his job if he simply writes off the adolescent as "cured" and forgets about him as soon as ten or 12 convulsions have apparently alleviated the depressive symptoms.

Despite its demonstrated efficacy in selected cases, electrotherapy remains controversial for at least two reasons. First, some psychiatrists believe, in the face of all evidence to the contrary, that there is no such thing as a biologic disorder called depressive illness, and that ECT represents, at worst, an assault on the patient and, at best, a roadblock in the way of the patient's psychologic resolution of the underlying problems, allegedly unconscious, which have caused the depression. Many scientific observations dating back to the 1930's refute these contentions,[3] and people who oppose ECT on these grounds fail to take this evidence into account. It is cruel to deny effective treatment to a depressed teenager who has failed to benefit from medication and whose extreme disorder of mood, and the disruption of physiologic function, thought processes, and social intercourse which accompany it, make insight psychotherapy impossible and at least temporarily irrelevant.

A second reason for opposition to electroconvulsive therapy is that it is over-used by some psychiatrists who apply it indiscriminantly to people with behavior disorders, hysteria, antisocial personality, anxiety neurosis, situational reactions, and so forth. The only thing good that can be said for such sloppy practice and such ignorance of psychiatric diagnosis or the proper place of ECT, is that at least those physicians are probably not failing to give ECT to the minority of patients who really need it.

Of course, ECT is also properly used in some schizophrenics and manics, as will be mentioned later. However, this chapter will not include a discussion of the specific techniques of ECT, for which the reader is referred elsewhere.[3]

Depressive illness is not preventable by any means now known, except perhaps in some cases of manic depressive illness, where prophylactic use of lithium may be indicated. However, early treatment of depression is certainly an attainable goal and can be "preventive" in a real sense—preventing an increase of severity, the necessity for hospitalization or ECT, and suicide. Everyone who works with teenagers should be alerted to early signs of depressive illness. And the patients themselves, once they have experienced an episode of depression, can recognize the symptoms of a subsequent episode much earlier and seek treatment before the illness becomes serious and disrupts their lives. In this way, the first episode of illness might have educational value for the patient, who can in the future benefit from knowledge gained during this distressing experience.

Suicidal Communication and Behavior

Considered by itself, the fact that a teenager has attempted suicide or made a serious suicidal communication tells little about him except that he probably has a psychiatric disorder. This is true even if the suicidal talk or action was precipitated by a stressful event. The doctor's duty to an adolescent exhibiting such behavior is to examine the act in its clinical and social context, just as he would any other symptom. Diagnosis is the principal clue to the psychiatric seriousness of a suicidal communication or attempt. For example, according to Robins and co-workers, persons with depressive illness and chronic alcoholism are those most likely to commit suicide.[4] Those with antisocial personality and hysteria, who form a substantial proportion of adolescent suicide attempters, rarely kill themselves. As mentioned in Chapter 5, an apparent triviality of circumstances preceding an attempt, and a lack of medically serious consequences, are not indications that a patient is not a serious suicidal risk.

When a physician is presented with a patient who has just attempted suicide, he must first determine whether a medical emergency exists. This is done by an assessment of the degree of severity of injury or intoxication resulting from the attempt. The doctor must also take a careful history from all persons available concerning exactly what the patient did to himself, so that a prediction can be made about the clinical course during the next few hours. For example, some medications (such as glutethimide) do not show their most potent toxic effects until some time after they are ingested. Alert patients have been released from emergency rooms after drug ingestion, only to lapse into coma after they have returned home. If there is any suspicion that the attempt might be medically serious, the adolescent should be seen by a physician competent to evaluate the emergency and able to admit the patient, if necessary, to a medical or surgical ward or intensive care unit. It should be stressed that even adolescents without serious psychiatric disorders may make medically serious suicide attempts. The fact that a drug ingestion or self-injury was inflicted by an immature, querulous teenager for obviously manipulative reasons should not prevent the doctor from suspecting that a medical emergency exists.

A complete psychiatric history and mental status examination is an indispensable part of the *immediate* evaluation of anyone who has just attempted suicide or seriously communicated his intentions to do so. There is no more propitious time for the physician to get a relevant history about the circumstances surrounding the attempt or communication and the clinical context in which it took place. Informants are usually on the scene, and the memories of events and symptoms are fresh in everyone's mind. The doctor should not be deterred by the fact that the patient, his relatives, and friends may be in great distress. The facts may be much more easily obtained at the time of the emergency than later, and a properly conducted psychiatric evaluation does not represent a callous intrusion on such an occasion. On the contrary, omission of such an examination at this time is an act of neglect, and can be most harmful to the patient.

If the adolescent presents with a suicide attempt or communication as the principal reason for his referral, this should usually be the first topic covered in the interview. He should be encouraged to give a detailed, spontaneous account of the events leading to the self-destructive behavior. If this history is complete, the examiner will find in it most important clues to the diagnosis and to the reasons for suicidal intent. A premature barrage of leading questions, however relevant ("Why did you do it?" "Are you depressed?"), can waste time, obstruct the adolescent's own account, and lead him to respond only in terms of the interviewer's expectations. For example, the author has found that teenagers are often reluctant to say that they took an overdose of pills *because* they had just had a broken date, or some other minor stress. But in a spontaneous account of the hour by hour events and symptoms leading to the suicide attempt, such information will usually emerge in its proper context. In this way the examiner is likely to learn about the patient's reasons for wanting to die, the degree of seriousness of the attempt or communication, the degree of persistence of death wishes, motives for attempting or talking about suicide at that particular time and place, expectations about rescue, hopes of changing the behavior of others, and so forth. All these facts must be learned if proper psychiatric treatment is to proceed. The interviewer must finally examine these subjects systematically by specific questioning after the patient has completed his own spontaneous history.

Although it is true that suicidal communications and attempts are psychiatric symptoms, they are nevertheless in a special category, since they are symptoms which the patient himself initiates. It makes sense, then, to assess the motivations and expectations preceding the patient's suicidal behavior, since such an assessment may provide important clues to diagnosis and management. If the suicidal behavior is recent, it is usually possible for the doctor to elicit such explanations of the timing and motivation for the behavior, even from psychotic patients whose reasons for wanting to die make sense only in the context of their delusions. For example, suppose that an adolescent who has never misbehaved and whose life has been free of external stress tells the interviewer that, after long consideration, he finally decided to attempt suicide when he was left alone and became more painfully aware than ever of his sinfulness and the hopelessness of his future. That patient would be altogether different, in terms of diagnosis and indicated treatment, from one who has a long history of antisocial behavior, is habitually manipulative of others, and tells the examiner that he attempted suicide because his girl friend left him, saying the act was carried out in the hopes that it would bring her back, although at the time he "really did not want to live." Of course, in order to arrive at a definite diagnosis and decide upon the treatment, the doctor will then need to conduct a systematic interview. But the spontaneous account of the most important circumstances leading to consultation may contain the most valuable leads to the psychopathology or social disruption for which the patient needs help.

Treatment of the patient who has attempted suicide or communicated his intent to do so depends upon the psychiatric diagnosis. But if the physician believes that the adolescent may kill himself, whatever his diagnosis, he should put him in a psychiatric hospital or see that adequate supervision is provided until the patient is no longer suicidal.

There is no fool-proof way to predict suicide, but there are several indications of serious risk which can lead the doctor to take precautions for his patient's protection. First, the patient should be asked if he wants to kill himself. An affirmative answer which does not appear to be a manipulative device or a taunt may be the most reliable indication of suicidal risk. The doctor should then ascertain if the patient has made specific plans to kill himself and if he has at his disposal the means to carry out his plans. Even in the absence of specific suicidal communication, the doctor should be alerted to the danger of a self-destructive act in an adolescent with depressed affect who sincerely affirms that he feels worthless, a burden to his family, thinks of death, and sees no future for himself. Questions should be asked about these items if the patient does not volunteer the information.

American studies of teenage suicides indicate that not only patients with depressive illness but also schizophrenics are the greatest risks. On the basis of these published reports and comparative studies of diagnostic labeling in Great Britain and the United States,[5] the author suspects that at least some of these "schizophrenics" would be called "depressed" or "schizoaffective" by the criteria of the current study. Nevertheless, the possibility remains that young schizophrenics (who may have prominent affective symptoms early in the course of a chronic illness) may be in danger of suicide. In any event, a patient with severe psychiatric disorder in which depressive affect is present and the process or content of thought is significantly disturbed should be considered a potential suicide risk until proven otherwise. Such extremely ill patients are often impervious to reassurance, inaccessible to interpersonal contact, and uninfluenced by changes for the better in their life circumstances. The doctor can often sense this ominous inaccessibility during the initial interview. If such a patient harbors suicidal plans, he may keep them to himself. Even if he expresses them, his reasons for wanting to die, based on firmly held delusions, may make it impossible for the physician or his family to change his mind by affection, exhortation or reassurance.

Mania

It is especially important to begin treatment for mania early in the course of the illness. If this is not done, there may be serious social consequences from the patient's poor judgment, hyperactivity, expansive mood, and irritability. Debts, ill-conceived and grandiose enterprises, embarrassing public behavior, indiscreet sexual promiscuity, alienation of associates, and disruption of family life are a partial list of complications of the illness. In addition, physical exhaustion is common by the time the patient reaches the doctor, and the majority of manic episodes are preceded or followed by depression.[6]

The difficulty about early intervention is that manic patients do not usually consider themselves sick or in need of treatment, and the family of the manic teenager may attribute the initial signs of mania, such as stubbornness and unwarranted exuberance, merely to vexing personality changes of adolescence. If the illness proceeds to the point of delusions and frenzied behavior, it is still unusual for the patient to initiate treatment for the first episode of mania. His family, worried about his state of mind, his unquenchable enthusiasm for unreasonable enterprises, his impatience, and his pugnacity, are the ones who seek help for him.

Once an adolescent's manic episode is well underway, it is difficult to treat him as an outpatient. This would require a great deal of time, firmness, and patience on the part of the family, and cooperation by the teenager. He must not only be persuaded that he is sick and in need of medication, but he will often be expected to take, exactly as prescribed, lithium carbonate, a drug with a narrow margin between minimum effective blood levels and toxic levels. All this may be too much to expect of the patient and his family, especially if they have no previous experience with mania, or if the episode is severe.

Hospitalization, then, is often desirable. Not only can the patient receive proper treatment which will shorten the illness but he can be protected from the consequences of his poor judgment. His aggressive encounters with all and sundry and his involvement in multiple enterprises can be curtailed. It is customary for manic patients to chafe at the restrictions placed upon them in the hospital, but the doctor should be cautioned against premature restoration of privileges—visitors, passes off the ward, phone privileges—or premature discharge from the hospital. The social restraint imposed by hospitalization, coupled with the appropriate use of medication, exerts a dampening effect on the patient's over-activity. The medical and nursing staff must be firm and patient in dealing with the provocations, threats, and manipulations of the manic teenager. They must recognize that this behavior is symptomatic of the illness, not characteristic of the patient's personality, and that it will pass if he remains in treatment. All this must be carefully explained to the family, whose cooperation is essential if therapy is not to be interrupted prematurely by their accession to the patient's demands for release.

Lithium carbonate has been established as an effective and safe treatment for mania, if there are no medical contraindications to its use and if blood levels are monitored. Current studies indicate that levels between 1.0 and 1.5 mEq./liter may be necessary to alleviate manic symptoms and prevent their recurrence.[7] Levels above 1.5 mEq./liter are inadvisable as they are associated with toxicity, and in a small minority of patients, usually elderly, serious poisoning and even death have been reported with moderately elevated blood levels.[8] The reader is referred to other work for detailed instructions of the use of lithium and discussion of possible mechanisms of its action.[9]

The beneficial effects of chlorpromazine and other phenothiazine drugs in episodes of mania have also been well demonstrated. This class of drugs is one of the safest used for treating psychiatric illnesses, and quite high doses, up to 2 gm. daily, have often been given to manic patients. The patients are more likely to complain of feeling "drugged" with chlorpromazine than with lithium given in therapeutic doses. But a phenothiazine may be necessary to control the symptoms of mania early in an episode, before lithium has had time to take effect, and in cases where there is extreme hyperactivity or combativeness, even while the patient has a therapeutic blood level of lithium.

Electrotherapy is effective in mania, although more treatments are usually required than for depression.[10] The author and most other psychiatrists at the Washington University Medical Center reserve ECT for those teenagers whose mania does not subside on medication or who are frenzied to the point of extreme exhaustion. Only one of the 11 manics in the current investigation received ECT during the study admission.

As mentioned in Chapter 4, in the controlled setting of the hospital the behavior of manics usually returns to normal before their mood and judgment do. This often leads the doctor to discharge the patient before he is well. Then he is faced with the necessity of readmitting his patient who had "rebounded" back into mania, or who has developed the depressive phase of the disorder. This cannot always be prevented, of course, but the physician can reduce the incidence of premature discharge by daily systematic interviews to ascertain the patient's mood, future plans, and current thought content. The doctor should especially ask about the particular delusions, grandiose expectations, or unjustifiable suspicions which the patient may have harbored when he was admitted. The fact that he may have stopped voicing these ideas spontaneously does not mean they are no longer present.

Even when an adolescent is apparently fully recovered before discharge, he should be maintained on medication and followed closely for a time after discharge. In the case of an isolated episode of mania, lithium or chlorpromazine may be tapered off and discontinued within a couple of months following discharge. But after that, close contact with the psychiatrist is necessary to insure that the remission is complete.

It has now been convincingly demonstrated that persons with chronic bipolar illness or repetitive episodes of mania or depression benefit from maintenance on lithium over a period of years.[11, 12] They have fewer, less severe, and briefer attacks; and they require significantly less hospitalization or ECT than they did before lithium maintenance was instituted or than they do after it is discontinued. Such prophylactic use of lithium is indicated in cooperative bipolar patients if they have had several episodes in the space of a few years. There are also indications that even in patients who have never had mania but who have cyclic attacks of depression (clearly demarcated from their usual state) may benefit from prophylactic lithium treatment.[12]

Once a patient has recovered from an attack of mania, the doctor should review the early signs and symptoms of that episode with him and his family. In this way prompt treatment, usually with lithium, can be reinstituted much earlier in the course of a future episode at a time when the patient is more likely to be cooperative. The symptoms can be brought under control more quickly and hospitalization avoided. Over the years, the author has been gratified that a number of his young patients, whom he saw during hospitalization for the first episode of mania, have learned to recognize their own particular early symptoms. For one patient it is early morning awakening, for another it is the onset of facial tics, for a third it is surges of erotic feelings for inappropriate people, and so forth. The development of long-term cooperativeness and reliability on the part of a patient depends to a great extent on how the psychiatrist handles the initial episode and its aftermath. If he spends time with the patient in supportive psychotherapy, builds a mutually trusting relationship after recovery, and explains the nature of the disorder insofar as it is understood, the physician may exert a substantial influence on his young patient's future response to recurrences of his illness.

Schizophrenia

The treatment of psychiatry's most vexing disorder, or group of disorders, classified under the diagnostic term, schizophrenia (see Chapter 6), was greatly advanced by two developments in the 1950's. Phenothiazines were introduced, and a change in mental hospitals' administrative policies resulted in greater attention to chronically ill patients, earlier discharge for schizophrenics, and more successful maintenance in the community. These last developments were stimulated, at least in part, by increases in public financial support for the training of psychiatrists, for research in mental disorders, and for enlargement of the cohort of psychiatric nursing personnel and other mental health professionals.

Nevertheless, the state of affairs where schizophrenia is concerned remains unsatisfactory. Investigators are in disagreement about appropriate subclassification of the disorder or disorders. The results of tests of hypotheses about causes, whether biologic, sociologic, or psychologic, have been disappointing so far. And except for those among the "schizoaffective" subgroup whose course of illness most closely resembles that of manic-depressive disease, the results of therapy are far from ideal.

There is probably no form of psychiatric treatment which has not been used in schizophrenia. Intensive psychotherapy, insulin coma, electrotherapy, sleep therapy, brain surgery, milieu therapy, massive doses of vitamins, and many other treatments have had their enthusiastic advocates. But, as of 1973, no form of treatment has been proven unequivocally effective in chronic schizophrenia except phenothiazines and butyrophenones. Double-blind, cross-over studies comparing such drugs with placebo, with other medications, and other forms of treatment, have repeatedly demonstrated their value.[2] They can reduce and often eliminate hallucinations, delusions, bizarre and antagonistic behavior, disruption of thought processes, and agitation. Even social withdrawal, which may be secondary to disorders of thought process or content, can be alleviated to an extent by these medications. Discontinuation of the medication often results in a recurrence of symptoms in the chronically ill schizophrenic, who may thus be destined to take the drug indefinitely if he is to remain out of the hospital and function with some degree of effectiveness.

Electroconvulsive therapy has proven helpful in those cases of acute onset which have a prominent affective component mixed with schizophrenic symptoms ("schizoaffective," or "schizophreniform" illness). As mentioned previously, a high proportion of such patients, perhaps half to two-thirds, may have a variant of manic-depressive illness. ECT has also been useful in catatonic patients, whose clinical picture is dominated by disorders of motility, such as posturing, immobility, or frenzied excitement. In some chronic patients, whose illnesses are characterized by delusions, hallucinations, or formal thought disorder, catatonic phases occasionally occur and present a crisis because the patient is not eating or is running about uncontrollably. In such cases, electrotherapy has been helpful in returning the patients to their habitual (and less threatening) clinical state, although it does not cure them.

The fact remains that the outcome of treatment in schizophrenia is probably determined more by the nature of the illness than by anything the physician does for the patient. There are good and bad prognostic signs whose importance over-rides the importance of any form of treatment. Vaillant[13] and other workers have studied these clinical features. In general, the more nearly the patient's course of illness, clinical picture, and family history resemble those of affective disorder, the more likely he is to recover. By contrast, a schizophrenic with poor prognostic features such as insidious onset, a withdrawn premorbid personality, and affective blunting may go on to deterioration and social incapacity despite the use of phenothiazines and the most assiduous personal attention to his case. But when a psychiatrist is called upon to treat a teenager with schizophrenia, he should not be deterred from vigorous therapy if poor prognostic signs are present. He should assume that he is dealing with a patient who may recover if treated properly.

First of all, it is important for the physician to establish a mutually trusting relationship with the patient and his family and to maintain this relationship during the course of therapy. This may be more important in the treatment of schizophrenia than of any other psychiatric disorder, in spite of the fact that the symptoms of schizophrenia are not alleviated by the development of such a relationship. It is important because the nature of the disorder must be explained to the family, not just at the beginning of treatment, but recurrently over the months or years of therapy. It is important because the teenager himself will need to trust his doctor in order to take the medicine in the dose prescribed. He will also need to confide in the doctor if the latter is to be of help to him in counseling. The necessity for this is paramount in the schizophrenic who is being treated as an outpatient. In the course of his everyday life he will be called upon to make decisions concerning school, job, and relationships with other people. Under even the most ideal circumstances of medication dosage, the patient's judgment may be distorted and he may be inclined to act on the basis of delusions. The risk of this is considerably reduced if he is willing to discuss his beliefs and plans with his therapist and if he feels secure enough to reveal the premises on which he bases his conclusions. Of course, some delusions and misjudgment will not be changed by anything the psychiatrist says, and he should not engage in fruitless arguments about fixed beliefs. The patient might interpret such controversy as evidence of rejection, ridicule or enmity. On the other hand, the psychiatrist can often, by gentle logic and suggesting alternative ways of viewing subjects, help the patient free himself of those delusions which are not so firmly held. Furthermore, the physician can often persuade the patient not to talk or behave publicly in a way that will make other people believe he is odd.

Many ambulatory schizophrenics have partial insight into the fact that some of the things they see, hear, think, or do are symptoms of a psychiatric disorder. Many, while not conceding that they are sick in any way, will acknowledge that well meaning people consider them nervous or peculiar. Still other schizophrenics, denying that they are ill and completely antagonistic to any people who suggest that they might be, will admit to "nervousness" or some other subjective symptom and will on that account agree to take phenothiazines and keep in touch with a psychiatrist.

The psychiatrist may be giving the medication because the patient hears voices and believes himself to be an object of hostile plots, whereas the patient may be taking the medicine because all this harrassment makes him nervous. What really matters is that he take the medicine. It is not the doctor's job to convince that schizophrenic patient to share his point of view entirely.

Delusions concerning the doctor or the medication are important to discover, because they are most likely to interfere with treatment. Trust of the physician and confidence in his therapy are seldom complete, and the physician must bear this in mind, even when the schizophrenic patient appears most friendly and open. The doctor should occasionally inquire about the patient's possible doubts concerning the treatment, side effects of the medication, advice given by the therapist, and so forth. Often simple explanation will set the patient's fears temporarily to rest.

Studies of medication-taking reveal that patients (whether they suffer from psychiatric or non-psychiatric disorders) seldom take oral medication exactly as it is prescribed all the time. The more times per day they are supposed to take medication, the less likely they are to adhere to a specific dosage schedule. If the patient is deluded or suspicious, or simply apathetic and preoccupied, he is even less likely to take his medication properly. When a schizophrenic fails to respond to phenothiazines, the doctor should first consider the possibility that he is not taking enough of the medicine. Even if he is in a hospital, it is easy for the patient to avoid swallowing tablets. Use of a liquid or injectable form of phenothiazine, administered by the nursing staff, usually avoids this problem. For outpatients, the injectable phenothiazines in an oil base, such as fluphenazine enanthate, can provide a sustained antipsychotic effect from one to four weeks, depending on the patient. The development of these products has been most helpful in the outpatient management of chronic schizophrenics.

The reader is referred elsewhere for discussions of the complications and side effects of antipsychotic drugs.[2] The author does not advocate the automatic use of antiparkinson drugs (benztropine mesylate, trihexphenidyl) along with phenothiazines, but reserves their use for those patients who develop extrapyramidal side effects. Even when such side effects are present early in the course of phenothiazine therapy, they may disappear after a time. So the physician should make periodic attempts to withdraw antiparkinson drugs while his patients are being maintained on phenothiazines.

If the schizophrenic adolescent fails to respond to phenothiazines, electroconvulsive therapy is indicated, unless such treatment has been adequately tried in the past and demonstrated to be of no benefit to that particular patient. In cases with acute onset, marked confusion, or the predominance of affective symptoms, it may be wise to use ECT first. The patient may be suffering from an atypical manic-depressive episode, in which case electrotherapy will be quicker, more effective, and approximately as safe as phenothiazines, while it is hastening the remission.

Antisocial Personality and Similar Disorders

The traditional therapies of psychiatry have contributed little, if anything, to the treatment of adolescents with a fully developed antisocial personality. Nothing the physician does *to* his sociopathic patient (medication, electrotherapy, etc.) will make him stop behaving badly for long. Of course, locking the patient in a hospital will temporarily interrupt the excesses of his antisocial activity. But this is only a temporary expedient, and such patients are able to be so disruptive in their behavior toward other patients and staff, even on a locked ward, that their presence there is soon unwelcome. Moreover, they are poor candidates for psychotherapy, as they usually lack the sustained motivation for change and the capacity to form meaningful relationships which are requisite for success in psychotherapy, individual or group, supportive or reconstructive.

As a consequence the psychiatrist and the sociopath usually shun each other's company, or have only brief contact, since they seldom have anything to offer one another. On the other hand, parents, school teachers, camp counselors, professionals in juvenile correction systems, and prison personnel do not enjoy the luxury of being able to avoid teenagers with antisocial personalities. It is they who are faced with the daily task of coping with the youngsters' misbehavior, trying to channel them into productive activity, or (if that fails) applying restraints which will prevent them from causing more trouble for themselves and other people.

Recently, Le Vine and Bornstein[14] have reviewed the literature on the treatment of antisocial personality and summarized its discouraging results. Under the circumstances, it makes more sense to talk about prevention of antisocial personality in children who have a prospect for developing the disorder, and the treatment of those adolescents who have a behavior disorder which is milder than antisocial personality and of those who are motivated to become socially productive. Even in those cases, physicians often play a smaller role than do parents, teachers, or counselors who work in special educational and training facilities.

Studies have shown that the risk for development of antisocial personality is probably increased for children who are aggressive and restless (including those with the fully developed hyperkinetic syndrome), especially if they behave in an antisocial, destructive manner before their teens.[15, 16] It is also increased in children whose parents have antisocial personality, drug addiction, or alcoholism; and in those whose homes have been broken by death or divorce and who suffer from lack of supervision or consistent discipline.[15]

The restlessness, short attention span, and learning disabilities so often encountered in children predisposed to antisocial personality lead to early problems in school. The child may respond to scholastic failure and reprimand by antagonistic behavior and truancy. In the manner of a vicious circle, failure and misbehavior may both increase until the child's or adolescent's academic career is terminated prematurely. This in turn may lead to idleness and trouble-making and to lower social and economic achievement later in life. By the time a psychiatrist sees a teenager who has experienced this process, the patient often has a durable sense of being a failure. This low self-esteem is an additional obstacle to the patient's improving his lot by sticking to difficult tasks and learning skills which will suit him for a socially and economically productive life. Moreover, such patients' feelings of tension and discouragement, as well as their risk-taking tendencies, often lead them to use excessive amounts of alcohol and drugs. These problems, even in the absence of illegal behavior and trouble with police, can undermine the development of a productive social role for the adolescent.

It follows from the above considerations that the hyperkinetic syndrome (which unlike sociopathy *is* often improved by drug therapy, specifically, the stimulants detroamphetamine and methylphenidate) should be treated early; that supervision and appropriate discipline should be given to children and adolescents who lack them; and that alternative learning situations should be provided for those youths who cannot adapt to standard educational and training institutions. In this category are tutoring programs and special schools or camps where youngsters can pursue activities which interest them and in which they can experience success in a productive endeavor, perhaps for the first time in their lives.

It should be said that success in these ventures can never be assured and that such an ideal program for preventing antisocial personality can be costly and time consuming, requiring a high teacher to pupil, or counselor to client, ratio. Although it has been demonstrated that childhood hyperkinesis, aggression, and antisocial behavior may lead to the development of sociopathy, and that discontinuation of school and poor supervision make a poor outcome more likely in such a child, there are as yet no data which show that the treatment of hyperkinesis prevents sociopathy, nor that improved supervision or special learning programs have a lasting effect on children at risk for the syndrome. The few controlled studies of treatment and education programs have had discouraging results (see Robins,[17] Le Vine and Bornstein,[14] and the Ahlstrom and Havighurst study of *400 Losers*[18]).

Nevertheless, common sense dictates that such methods of prevention should be tried when they are practical. If a child is exposed to habitual neglect or abuse, and a better situation in a foster home or special school is available, it should be provided. (Unfortunately, a better situation is often *not* available, especially to the children of poor families who may need help most.) Counseling for parents and adolescents with respect to the problems of everyday life together; exploration in psychotherapy of the roots of conflict arising between teenagers and their parents, teachers, or employers; zealous searching for suitable schools or alternative programs: all these methods will be tried by the interested psychiatrist whose patients give some evidence of motivation for change.

Hysteria*

This disorder, as described by Guze and others[19] (see Chapter 7), is apparently related to antisocial personality,[20] although its determinants are less well understood than are those of the latter syndrome. Since girls with hysteria are frequently seen by non-psychiatric physicians, the latter are theoretically in a position to reduce some of its complications—doctor-shopping, over-medication, unnecessary hospitalization and surgery, manipulation of families and schools by symptoms, and so forth. The physician must be able to recognize hysteria when he encounters it, and willing to maintain the communication with patients, parents, teachers, counselors and other physicians which can result in the saving of the family's time and money. The results of insight psychotherapy for hysterics have been quite discouraging.

Phobias

Phobias (irrational fears) often begin in childhood or adolescence.[21] When presented with a teenager who complains of phobias, the physician should first rule out the possibility that his patient suffers from affective disorder or schizophrenia. If he does, then treatment of the primary disorder is indicated.

Uncomplicated phobias should be discussed with the patient to see if they are manifestations of obvious life conflicts or specific, correctable situations. If they are, they may be amenable to treatment by brief psychotherapy or family counseling. In more resistant cases, long-term psychotherapy to uncover unconscious conflicts has been much less effective than behavior therapy, by such methods as relaxation and systematic desensitization described by Wolpe[22] and Marks.[21] The therapist can

* Hysteria is here distinguished from conversion symptoms. The latter are unexplained neurologic symptoms which often appear in hysteria, but also in many other psychiatric disorders, as well as in neurologic illnesses which may be in their early stages and therefore not yet diagnosable.

continue to discuss relevant personal problems with his patient during a portion of the interview, while reserving another part of each session for the relaxation-desensitization program. Psychotherapy and behavior therapy are not mutually exclusive.

Behavior therapy is much more effective for patients with isolated specific phobias than for those with widespread phobias accompanied by disabling anxiety. The latter syndrome, called "agoraphobia" by Marks[21] and the "phobic-anxiety-depersonalization" state by Roth,[23] often begins in adult life and is extremely resistant to any mode of treatment.

Obessive-Compulsive Neurosis

This disorder is dominated by persistent and recurrent thoughts (obsessions), or actions, which are accompanied by feelings of compulsion or irresistibility. Patients commonly recognize their symptoms as illogical and try to resist thinking the obsessive thoughts and performing the compulsive acts. A number of longitudinal studies of this illness have recently been summarized by Goodwin, *et al.*[24] Most patients with milder varieties of this, whether with chronic or intermittent symptoms, probably do not seek psychiatric assistance. Of those who do see psychiatrists, the majority have transient or moderate disability. But a significant minority, perhaps as many as 25% to 40%, experience persistent disability, regardless of the therapy used. Psychiatrists have employed a variety of techniques for treating obsessive-compulsives—insight psychotherapy, relaxation-desensitization for phobic symptoms, antidepressants when depressive symptoms supervene, ECT, and so forth. Recent literature, especially from Great Britain, has added support to the use of leukotomy for chronically disabled cases, almost always middle-aged adults, who have failed to respond to all other forms of treatment over many years.

There has been a notable dearth of prospective studies of children and adolescents with severe obsessive-compulsive neurosis, and a lack of large scale studies of first-degree relatives of such patients in any age group. There are reports of teenagers who had well established obsessive-compulsive neurosis and whose symptoms later remitted. On the other hand, a small minority of obsessive-compulsive youngsters have later developed schizophrenia. The possibility of a relationship between these two disorders in some cases is being investigated by Reich at Washington University in a longitudinal and family study.[25]

Anxiety Neurosis

Anxiety neurosis is said to occur in 5% to 10% of the population.[26] This syndrome begins at an early age and tends to be chronic but nondisabling in the great majority. Nervousness and easy fatiguability are common complaints. "Anxiety attacks"—with tachycardia, chest pain, hyperventilation, and at times tetany and syncope—may be provoked by emotionally significant stress or may occur without discoverable cause. The etiology of this syndrome is unknown. Psychodynamic theories of its origin, dating back to Freud, remain untested; and the intriguing study of Pitts and McClure,[27] demonstrating an abnormality of lactate metabolism in the production of anxiety attacks, needs replication on larger populations of patients.

The adolescent with anxiety neurosis, in which physical symptoms play so large a role, commonly believes himself to be suffering from cardiac or respiratory disease. After an appropriate medical work-up, the physician can firmly reassure his young patient and the family that this is not the case. An explanation of anxiety neurosis is then in order, and the patient should understand that it is not life threatening. Patients with this syndrome may become anxious in situations which would not provoke this response in others. Accordingly, supportive psychotherapy and reassurance may be in order, as well as treatment with minor tranquilizers like diazapam and chlordiazepoxide. Anxiety neurotics are also likely to develop phobias and a fearful avoidance of situations which have in the past been associated with anxiety attacks. In these instances, the illness can become disabling, restricting social and occupational activities. Behavior therapy should then be undertaken, just as in phobic neurosis, and if this is successful the patient may be freed of the restriction imposed by his fears. In addition, sometimes a substantial amount of realistic self-doubt underlies the phobias of adolescents. They are, after all, facing new situations in school, in career choice, and in sexual relationships. They should have the opportunity to discuss these fears, explore their underlying bases, and receive factual information and appropriate reassurance in counseling.

Sexual Maturation and Problems

This is most properly a subject for inclusion in a volume on the normal development of adolescents. A few aspects of sexuality will be considered here, since psychiatrists and counselors are frequently consulted on such matters by their teenage patients.

First of all, the counselor of adolescents should make himself knowledgeable about matters of sexual development and behavior and be free of judgmental rigidity on the subject. Masters and Johnson,[28] Lief,[29] and others have pointed out that, in general, medical schools do not adequately cover the subjects of sexual development and disorders. Their graduates then go into practice, and whatever specialty they pursue, they are soon confronted by many patients with sexual problems. The "fund" of knowledge at their command is too often confined to their own sexual experience and bits of information picked up as clinical anecdotes.

Many adolescents' anxieties about their sexual feelings and behavior can be allayed by providing them with factual information after the counselor has elicited accounts of their specific fears, self-doubts, or social awkwardness.

Atypical sexual behavior—homosexuality, transvestism, transsexualism, fetishes, exhibitionism, voyeurism, and so forth—occurs in the absence of psychiatric illness, but may appear in some disorders. For example, sexual deviation may be present in adolescents with antisocial personality; a depressive symptom complex may develop in homosexuals, particularly after the rupture of important relationships[30]; and some forms of unusual sexual activity may have the characteristics of a compulsion which the patient seeks unsuccessfully to resist.

As a rule, sociopaths do not seek psychiatric treatment for anything at all, much less for sexual activity that is pleasurable to them, and efforts to change their behavior in this respect are doomed to failure.

Teenagers who develop depressive symptoms after the rupture of a homosexual relationship may seek treatment to alleviate their grief, not to change their sexual orientation. It is true that the degree of discomfort engendered by their loss may cause them to regret for a time that they are homosexual. They may request help in "going straight," only to lose their motivation for this change after they have recovered from their depression.

Teenagers who are neither sociopathic nor depressed and who seek help for socially condemned sexual behavior that they feel unable to resist (exhibitionism, pedophilia, etc.), often do so only after they have been reported to the police. Juvenile courts commonly refer such adolescents for psychiatric treatment after the first arrest. The youths then find themselves caught between their impulses for forbidden sexual behavior and the probability that a second or third arrest will result in punishment by legal authorities. Their desire for the change in behavior may be dependent upon the legal threat confronting them, and that may serve as sufficient motivation for successful treatment, for at least as long as the threat lasts.

Of course, many adolescents with no psychiatric disorder and no threat of court action hanging over them may seek psychiatric help in order to stop or diminish sexually deviant activity and the desire for such activity. They are usually also motivated to experience or increase hetero-erotic feelings and behavior toward peers.

The author rarely recommends that a teenager stop engaging in gratifying sexual behavior that is neither harming other people nor putting the adolescent himself in danger. But if a patient seeks to stop such activity, for whatever motive, the author attempts to help him. This involves detailed inquiry into the possible reasons for his current sexual orientation and behavior and exploration of the consequences of the behavior—pleasure, guilt, punishment, etc. Evaluation also involves inquiry into reasons for the adolescent's disinterest, fear, or disgust concerning heterosexual activity. No certain proof about causes can be expected from such exploration, but working theories about the roots and goals of the behavior can be formulated and may be helpful in the course of subsequent counseling. Discussions in psychotherapy will range far beyond sexual matters and will cover such topics as self-esteem, non-sexual relationships with other people, scholastic and job problems, general goals for the future, and so on. The patient's goals may change in the course of therapy. It is not unusual for a teenager with, for example, strong homosexual feelings to enter psychotherapy for the purpose of getting rid of these feelings and becoming heterosexual. He may later decide that other problems are of greater concern to him and concentrate on them instead. He may, on occasion, come to accept his homosexuality as inevitable after strenuous efforts to change, ridding himself of guilt.

No control studies have proven that psychotherapy is effective in changing deviant sexual behavior, but this does not mean that it does not work in some cases. Nor does this prevent psychiatrists from offering psychotherapy to these patients, who may be benefited by counseling with respect to other problems, even if their sexual proclivities remain unchanged.

The effects of behavior therapy on sexual deviation are easier to measure in controlled experiments than are those of psychotherapy. A number of reports indicate some success for aversion therapy, in which the therapist and patient systematically arrange for sexual excitement from the stimulus (a fetish, a homosexual photograph, fantasy of exhibitionism, etc.) to be immediately accompanied by an unpleasant sensation (pain, nausea, etc.). After courses of such treatment, patients have reported diminution in the intensity and frequency of sexual arousal by the specific objects or fantasies used in the therapy. Many therapists make reinforcement of heterosexual feelings an integral part of the treatment. This can be done, for example, if relief from the unpleasant sensation is immediately accompanied by a heterosexual stimulus. Behavior therapists stress the importance of technique and of the specificity and timing of various stimuli. Aversive conditioning cannot be expected to work if it is done haphazardly, and the reader is referred elsewhere for descriptions of techniques.[31]

As time passes after the completion of a course of aversion therapy, patients tend to experience a gradual return of their deviant symptoms and diminution of heterosexual feelings. Subsequent courses of behavior therapy may then be indicated. As with relaxation-desensitization therapy for phobias, aversive conditioning can be accompanied by psychotherapy.

The two different forms of therapy should take place during separate portions of each treatment session.

The therapist and patient should not be discouraged by the fact that a combination of behavior therapy and psychotherapy will not altogether extinguish deviant tendencies and replace them with hetero-erotic strivings. Even partial success in treatment may remove a great burden from a patient and enable him to pursue a happier and more productive life.

It has been shown that male homosexuals and transsexuals have a high incidence of effeminacy in childhood.[30] Green *et al.*[32] have advocated the treatment of very young effeminate boys by a program of behavior modification designed to discourage feminine behavior and reinforce masculine behavior, encouraging it partly through greater contact and identification with masculine adult males. He hopes that by this means the boys will avoid the personal stress and social complications in store for many homosexuals and transsexuals in our society. Of course, only a large scale longitudinal study will demonstrate whether such a preventive program is effective.

Anorexia Nervosa

This interesting disorder predominantly affects teenage girls or young adult women. It commonly begins with weight loss and amenorrhea, either of which may come first. It is accompanied by peculiar preoccupations about food and eating, desire for excessive thinness, and fear or extreme discomfort concerning weight gain. The patients are often quite physically active despite their considerable emaciation. "Anorexia" is not always an accurate term, as many patients profess to have voracious appetites. They may resist attempts to make them gain weight by lying, hiding food, and vomiting. Their stubborn denial of the gravity of their state, coupled with the parents' extreme frustration and concern, inevitably lead to conflict in the family. This has usually become quite prominent by the time the psychiatrist sees the patient.

We restrict this diagnosis to people who have an onset before age 25, and we exclude those who have a preexisting psychiatric disorder, such as depression or schizophrenia, in which extreme weight loss may also occur. When anorexia nervosa is defined in this way, it appears to be a well delimited syndrome in its own right, not a variant or early phase of some other illness. Follow-up studies show a range of outcomes—death from emaciation or its complications in up to 15%, recovery in some, and in others continued thinness to a less extreme degree, subsequent depression or anxiety in the absence of weight loss, continued menstrual disorders in many, and frigidity in many. The few family history studies and family studies fail to link anorexia nervosa convincingly with other psychiatric syndromes.[33] Metabolic and endocrinologic studies of the disorder, many of whose symptoms suggest pituitary or hypothalamic dysfunction, have been complicated by the fact that cachetic patients develop metabolic abnormalities secondary to their emaciation. Halmi and her associates at the University of Iowa have undertaken such studies with recently developed methods.[34] Their metabolic investigations of sick and recovered patients are being accompanied by follow-up and family studies of a large cohort of people with anorexia nervosa seen at that medical center since the 1930's. Such efforts may in time reveal the essential nature of this syndrome.

In the present state of our knowledge, treatment of adolescent girls with anorexia nervosa should have the primary goal of weight gain, and concomitant resolution of personal and family problems, whether those problems preceded the weight loss or were consequences of it. Every form of treatment has been tried with anorexia nervosa. Insight psychotherapy, antidepressants, and electroconvulsive therapy have not been demonstrated to be successful. The author advocates hospitalization and restriction of privileges during the first phase of treatment and the institution of a graduated system of increased privileges and rewards for weight gain until the patient has achieved her normal weight. These girls usually like to be well groomed and physically active, and they may be gregarious. Permission to fix their hair, use makeup, wear attractive clothes, have visitors, and leave their rooms, the ward, or the hospital, may be made contingent upon gaining a specified amount of weight each day. Some physicians couple this program with a sedating dose of a tranquilizer, for example, chlorpromazine. The amount of drug is gradually decreased as the patient gains weight, enabling her to engage in more and more of the activities she enjoys.

Usually the patient and the family question and resist such restrictive treatment at times during its course. The physician should explain the rationale behind his treatment and the dangers of anorexia nervosa. In addition, he should discuss with the patient and her parents the specific conflicts that arise in the family. Those discussions should continue after weight gain is achieved, since interpersonal discord may undermine the success of therapy.

It is common for patients to gain weight in the hospital and lose it again after discharge. Readmission is then advisable, and the treatment program should be repeated. In cases of refusal to eat under any circumstances, cautious tube feeding has been advocated by some writers, although others have warned of its dangers, for example, vomiting, aspiration, and pneumonia or asphyxia.

Of course, success is never assured in the treatment of anorexia nervosa. But the dangers of the disorder call for vigorous, prolonged, and repeated efforts on the part of physicians and nursing staffs; otherwise therapy will not have had a real trial, and the patient may die by default.

Alcohol and Drug Abuse

If alcohol or drug abuse by a teenager occurs only in the course of depression, mania, schizophrenia, or schizoaffective disorder, then this may cease to be a problem after adequate treatment of the primary condition. More commonly, however, such abuse arises in disorders for which there is no effective somatic therapy: antisocial personality, hysteria, and other (less well defined) personality disorders. And excess drinking or drug-taking may arise in teenagers who were previously well.

In this author's experience there is no sure way for parents to prevent their child from drinking or using drugs. They owe it to the youngster to be informed themselves and provide specific information about the dangers of various substances and the risks of intravenous administration of anything. And they owe it to him to keep informed about his associates and activities, to know of his whereabouts, and to avoid giving him a large and regular supply of unearned money. They should have established rules about performance of domestic and scholastic responsibilities, general behavior, curfew, and areas where their child is or is not permitted to go. These rules should have a rational basis and should be appropriate for the age, emotional stability, and maturity of the teenager. Such clearly understood rules may to some extent serve as a deterrent to drug and alcohol abuse, as well as other forms of deviant behavior. Unfortunately, the adolescent who most needs rules is most likely to question them and push beyond their boundaries, regardless of the fact that they may be rational, in his best interest, and not the products of parental over-concern or sheltering.

There is also no sure way for parents to know whether their teenager is taking drugs, unless they catch him doing it, unless he tells them, or unless he develops unmistakable toxic symptoms. Such "soft" signs in the early teens as personal sloppiness, laziness, loss of interest in school, and the adaptation of current fads of clothing and hair style may have no significance at all with respect to drugs or alcohol.

The vast majority of adolescents who use illicit drugs or alcohol never come to a physician's attention. The psychiatrist and the drug or alcohol abuser may first cross each other's path as a result of acute intoxication—the overdose of a sedative, or a bad trip from a psychedelic drug. After recovery from this episode, the patient should be offered counseling assistance, although there is a good chance that he will not follow this advice.

There is no evidence that any treatment ever devised will make a teenager stop drinking too much or taking too many drugs. In serious abusers the psychologic or physical need for the substances they are taking, usually more than one substance, may override warnings, lectures, insight, and a succession of disastrous consequences of abuse. The author has known many adolescents who passed through a phase of alcoholic and drug excess and stopped because of expense, unpleasant side effects, or their dissatisfaction with an unproductive life. However, it is rare for a patient to attribute his abstinence to psychiatric intervention.

Most therapists treating youths with those problems strive for the stabilization of the home and school environment, when possible, and maintain frequent contact with their patients to facilitate the discussion of personal issues. Disulfiram (Antabuse) may be of help in the alcoholic teenager who understands its side effects, wants to use it, and is willing to maintain regular contact with his therapist. In counseling, lectures about the evils of drink and dope are not useful. Specific information about the effects of the substances should be given if the therapist ascertains that the patient does not already know it. That may help. But, unfortunately, most adolescents who take drugs regard their own experience as the only reliable indicator of a drug's physical, psychologic, and social effects.

Chronic abuse of sedating drugs, such as the short and intermediate acting barbiturates and some minor tranquilizers can result in a state of physical dependence. Withdrawal of such substances should be gradual to prevent agitation, seizures, and delirium. Ewing and Bakewell have provided helpful information about successful withdrawal procedures.[35]

When amphetamine abuse results in a state resembling paranoid schizophrenia—with delusions of persecution, visual or auditory hallucinations, agitation, and belligerence, usually in a clear state of consciousness—the patient should be hospitalized and amphetamines withdrawn. Phenothiazines are indicated for this syndrome, and the patient usually recovers within a week or two. In a few patients, the symptoms persist for many weeks or months, or recur, raising the possibility that these people have schizophrenia independent of their drug abuse, or that the drug caused a persistent psychiatric disorder. Of course, a common cause of symptom recurrence is covert resumption of amphetamine abuse, which the patient may deny.

Narcotic addiction in the United States is currently being widely treated by maintenance on methadone. Early positive reports have indicated success in keeping a substantial portion of heroin addicts free of the latter drug and working productively at jobs. But reports of abuse of methadone, also an addicting substance, and the appearance of that drug in the illicit market raise questions about its long-term usefulness in the fight against heroin addiction. Long-term follow-up studies of addicts treated with methadone must be completed, and their results compared with results of such studies as those of Vaillant,[36] who has published an excellent follow-up of narcotic addicts first treated before methadone was widely introduced.

SOME CONSIDERATIONS ABOUT PSYCHOTHERAPY WITH ADOLESCENTS

Earlier sections of this chapter include remarks about psychotherapy, but further discussion is in order here.

Contact between a physician in any specialty and a patient should be psychotherapeutic, regardless of the type of disorder from which the patient suffers. That is, the physician should acquire an understanding of the major personal issues of his patient's life and of the interaction among life circumstances, emotions, and symptoms. In addition, as treatment of any type proceeds the doctor should continue to supply the patient with information about his illness. In turn, the physician should encourage his patient to keep him informed about important developments in his personal life, and he should function as a counselor when it is appropriate. The author has known surgeons and internists whose treatment of patients was more psychotherapeutic in these respects than that of many psychiatrists. Some of the latter are guilty of rigidity, insensitivity, and unwarranted haste in dealing with matters that fall outside the category of target symptoms.

It stands to reason, then, that psychotherapy in this broad sense of the word should be part of the treatment of any psychiatric disorder, even those syndromes for which psychotherapy is not useful by itself, such as schizophrenia, mania, and severe depressive illness, where somatic therapies play a crucial role.

For some patients, psychotherapy is the primary or only mode of treatment. This includes those who need counseling for specific life crises, those with mild disorders not susceptible to somatic therapy, and those whose personalities habitually lead them into difficulty, resulting in frequent disruption of their personal relationships and their performance at school or work. Psychotherapy for these patients is not the special province of psychiatrists. Although controlled studies of psychotherapy are difficult if not impossible to do, it is the author's impression that intelligent, imaginative, and well trained psychologists, social workers, and other counselors do as well as many psychiatrists, often better.

Psychotherapy must start with a systematic evaluation of the teenager and his family and the important events of his life, past and present. The sections at the beginning of this chapter dealing with preparation of the counselor, initial evaluation, substance of the first interview, and immediate treatment plans, outline the authors' views on this most crucial part of the therapeutic process.

If psychotherapy is to be an important part of an adolescent's treatment, the patient himself must have, or soon acquire, motivation for it. If he is in his early teens, or if he comes for treatment primarily at the instigation of others, his motivation for treatment may be tenuous at the beginning. The therapist should keep this in mind, for the patient may be reluctant to admit it, even if he is asked. An adolescent's motivation may be further reduced or altogether destroyed if the therapist adopts a rigid attitude or resorts to lecturing. If is doubtful that he will say anything in a lecture which the patient has not heard before from some other adult in authority.

At the outset, the therapist should explain the purposes of psychotherapy and the methods of accomplishing them. In general, these purposes will be to discover the adolescent's own goals, explore with him the feasibility of reaching them, and discuss the means of fulfilling those of his goals which seem realistic. The method of accomplishing these purposes is by talking about relevant issues in the past, present, and future. At the heart of motivation for psychotherapy is the adolescent's desire to change something about himself, the way he thinks, feels, or acts. If he does not want to change, psychotherapy will turn out to be a waste of time and money. Self-understanding, and the development of a relationship with the therapist are means to an end, never ends in themselves. If both the therapist and patient do not realize that, their mutual efforts will probably be of no benefit.

The author has not found that the principles and techniques of psychotherapy with adolescents are fundamentally different from those of psychotherapy with adults. However, there are some important distinctions between teenage and adult patients which should be kept in mind by therapists working with the younger age group. First, compared to an adult, an adolescent is more likely to have entered therapy at someone else's insistence. The resentment that might have arisen because of this can get in the way of the teenager's regarding psychotherapy as his own endeavor. He might persist in regarding the therapist as an agent for parents, school, juvenile court, etc., rather than his own employee. Second, because of the age difference between teenagers and psychiatrists, they are even more likely than adult patients to regard their therapists as authority figures. Third, since most adolescents know less about life than adults, the psychiatrists treating them are more often called upon to impart specific information and advice. The therapist should remember, however, that what he considers information the teenager may regard as preaching. Fourth, parents are in a position to facilitate or sabotage the results of psychotherapy with adolescents, especially younger teenagers. For this reason, periodic interviews with the parents are often indicated to help them understand and modify their own behavior toward their children. In addition, group conferences with a family may become an occasional or exclusive method of psychotherapy in selected cases. In this way the therapist, patient, and parents may better understand the nature of the family's interaction, increase productive communication, and decrease behavior that leads to conflicts and perpetuates the teenager's problems. Finally, adolescents change more rapidly than adults, not with respect to the evolution of specific psychiatric illnesses, but with respect to social maturity, interests, and physical and intellectual activity. It is this quality which makes psychotherapy with teenagers especially absorbing for the professional who is interested in watching young people grow, as well as in helping to relieve their suffering and the suffering of their families.

REFERENCES

1. Clayton, P. J., Halikas, J. A., and Maurice, W. L. The depression of widowhood. Br. J. Psychiatry *120:* 71–77, 1972.
2. Klein, D. F., and Davis, J. M. *Diagnosis and Drug Treatment of Psychiatric Disorders.* Baltimore, Williams & Wilkins Co., 1969.
3. Kalinowsky, L. B., and Hoch, P. H. *Somatic Treatments in Psychiatry.* New York, Grune and Stratton, Inc., 1961.
4. Robins, E., Murphy, G. E., Wilkinson, R. H., Jr., Gassner, S., and Kayes, J. Some clinical considerations in the prevention of suicide based on a study of 134 successful suicides. Am. J. Public Health *49:* 888–899, 1959.
5. Kendall, R. E., Cooper, J. E., Gourlay, A. J., Copeland, J. R. M., Sharpe, L., and Gurland, B. L. Diagnostic criteria of American and British psychiatrists. Arch. Gen. Psychiatry *25:* 123–130, 1971.
6. Winokur, G., Clayton, P. J., and Reich, T. *Manic Depressive Illness.* St. Louis, C. V. Mosby., 1969.
7. Prien, R. F., Caffy, E. M., Jr., and Klett, C. J. Relationship between serum lithium level and clinical response in acute mania treated with lithium. Br. J. Psychiatry *120:* 409–414, 1972.
8. Schou, M., Amdisen, A., Trap-Jensen, J. Lithium poisoning. Am. J. Psychiatry *125:* 520–527, 1968.
9. Gattozzi, A. A. *Lithium in the Treatment of Mood Disorders.* Washington, National Clearinghouse for Mental Health Information, N.I.M.H., Publication No. 5033, 1970.
10. Schiele, B. C., and Schneider, R. A. The selective use of electroconvulsive therapy in manic patients. Dis. Nerv. Ssyt. *10:* 291, 1949.
11. Baastrup, P. C., Paulsen, J. C., Schou, M., Thompsen, K., and Amdisen, A. Prophylactic lithium: double-blind discontinuation in manic-depressive and recurrent depressive disorders. Lancet *2:* 326–330, 1970.
12. Coppen, A., Noguera, R., Bailey, J., Burns, B. H., Swani, M. S., Hare, E. H., Gardner, R., and Maggs, R. Prophylactic lithium in affective disorders. Lancet *2:* 275–279, 1971.
13. Vaillant, G. E. Prospective prediction of schizophrenic remission. Arch. Gen. Psychiatry *11:* 509–518, 1964.
14. Le Vine, W. R., and Bornstein, P. E. Is the sociopath treatable? The contribution of psychiatry to a legal dilemma. Washington University Law Quarterly, Number 4, 1973.

15. Robins, L. N. *Deviant Children Grown Up*. Baltimore, Williams & Wilkins Co., 1966.
16. Mendelson, W., Johnson, N., and Stewart, M. A. Hyperactive children as teenagers. J. Nerv. Ment. Dis. *153:* 273–279, 1971.
17. Robins, L. N. The evaluation of psychiatric services for children in the U.S.A. Proceedings of the World Psychiatric Association, Second Symposium on Psychiatric Epidemiology, 1972.
18. Ahlstrom, W. M., and Havighurst, R. J. *400 Losers: Deliquent Boys in High School.* San Francisco, Jossey-Bass, Inc., 1971.
19. Perley, M., and Guze, S. B. Hysteria—the stability and usefulness of clinical criteria. N. Engl. J. Med. *266:* 421–426, 1962.
20. Guze, S. B., Woodruff, R. A., and Clayton, P. J. Hysteria and antisocial behavior: further evidence of an association. Am. J. Psychiatry *127:* 957–960, 1971.
21. Marks, I. M. *Fears and Phobias.* London, Heinemann Medical, 1969.
22. Wolpe, J. *Psychotherapy by Reciprocal Inhibition.* Stanford, Stanford University Press, 1958.
23. Roth, M. The phobic anxiety-depersonalization syndrome and some general aetiological problems in psychiatry. J. Neuropsychiatry *1:* 293, 1960.
24. Goodwin, D. W., Guze, S. B., and Robins, E. Follow-up studies in obsessional neurosis. Arch. Gen. Psychiatry *20:* 182–187, 1969.
25. Reich, T. Personal communication (by permission).
26. Cohen, M. E. Neurocirculatory asthenia. Med. Clin. North Am. 1343–1364, 1949.
27. Pitts, F. N., Jr., and McClure, J. N., Jr. Lactate metabolism in anxiety neurosis. N. Engl. J. Med. *277:* 1329–1336, 1967.
28. Masters, W. H., and Johnson, V. E. *Human Sexual Inadequacy.* Boston, Little, Brown and Co., 1970.
29. Lief, H. I. What medical schools teach about sex. Bull. Tulane Univ. Med. Fac. *22:* 161–168, 1963.
30. Saghir, M. T., and Robins, E. *Male and Female Homosexuality.* Baltimore, Williams & Wilkins Co., 1973.
31. Feldman, M. P., and MacCulloch, J. F. The application of anticipatory avoidance learning to the treatment of homosexuality. I Theory, technique, and preliminary results. Behav. Res. Ther. *2:* 165–183, 1965.
32. Green, R., Newman, L. E., and Stoller, R. J. Treatment of boyhood "transsexualism." Arch. Gen. Psychiatry *26:* 213–217, 1972.
33. Theander, S. Anorexia nervosa: a psychiatric investigation of 94 female patients. Acta Psychiat. Scand., Supp. 214, 1970.
34. Halmi, K. A. Personal communication.
35. Ewing, J. A., and Bakewell, W. E. Diagnosis and management of depressant drug dependence. Am. J. Psychiatry *123:* 909–917, 1967.
36. Vaillant, G. E. A 20-year follow-up of New York narcotic addicts. Arch. Gen. Psychiatry *29:* 237–246, 1973.

Appendix I

Adolescent interview

Identifying Information

Date of interview:
Name of interviewer:
Name of patient (including maiden name):
Study number:
Renard admission number:
Barnes chart number:
Date of admission:
Birth date:
Age at last birthday:
Address:
Phone number:
Sex:
Race:
Current marital status:
Religion:
Full name of attending doctor (if not private, put "Staff"):
Name of parents, foster parents, or guardian (specify relationship):
Address of parents (or etc.):
Phone number of parents (or etc.):
Name of spouse:
Address of spouse:
Spouse's phone number:
At least two other adult relatives:
  Names:
  Relationship:
  Address:
Informant's name:
  Address:
  Phone number:
  Relationship:
  Length of time known patient:
  Frequency of contact:

Present Illness

Why are you in the hospital (patient's own reason)?
Why is he (or she) in the hospital (informant's reason)?
Chronologic account of present illness (use dates):
Patient's account (extensive and detailed history recorded here):
Informants' accounts (extensive and detailed history recorded here):
What was the first sign of this trouble? (If patient has used a specific term, like "depression," use that term in the question.)
When was that (date)?
Since then have you seen a doctor for this? Have you seen a psychiatrist, other doctor, minister or any kind of counselor or advisor?
How often?
Have you been taking any medicine or other kind of treatment?
What?
How often?
How much?
(At this point, review the "present illness" with the patient or informant, reading the essentials to him, and ask)
Is there anything else important that you haven't mentioned?
Have you ever had trouble like this before?
Tell me about it (dates).
Date of onset:
Symptoms and course:
Treatment:
What?
By whom?
Where?
Outcome:
Date of recovery:
Have you ever had any *other* kind of trouble with nervousness, depression, heavy drinking, nervous breakdown, in trouble at school or with the police? (Ask items *slowly,* with a pause after each.)
Tell me about it:
Date of onset:
Symptoms and course:
Treatment:
What?
By whom?
Where?
Outcome:
Date of recovery:
Again list the date of onset of *this episode.*

(From the information received so far check which *one* of these statements is true.)

— Before the date of onset above the patient never had any kind of psychiatric problems at all. Elaborate if appropriate:

— Before the date of onset the patient had at least one previous episode of the same type of psychiatric difficulty which cleared up completely. Elaborate if appropriate:

— Before the date of onset the patient had previous psychiatric symptoms of the same type which were chronic, although they may or may not have fluctuated in intensity. Elaborate if appropriate:

— Before the date of onset the patient had at least one previous episode of a different type of psychiatric illness which cleared up completely.

— Before the date of onset the patient had previous psychiatric symptoms of a different type which were chronic, although they may or may not have fluctuated in intensity.

Personal History

Ask the *patient:*

Tell me about your life, what kind of person you have been, the things that have happened to you and the things you have done, from as far back as you remember:

(Record important points verbatim.)

What are your plans for the future?

Why are you interested in this (in these things)?

Ask the *informant:*

Tell me about his (her) life, the kind of person he (she) is, the things he (she) has done and the things that have happened to him (her):

(Record important points verbatim.)

What sort of future have you hoped for for him (her)?

Have your hopes for him (her) changed?

What sort of future do you expect for him (her)?

What are your reasons for expecting this?

Have your expectations changed during his (her) life?

Ask patient and informant:

At this time do you feel you are (her or she is) different from your (his or her) usual self?

If so, please explain (1) in what way you are (he or she is) different and (2) when the difference was first noticeable and (3) what was the first thing which happened which made you aware of the difference (number paragraphs 1, 2 and 3). Then specify under paragraph "4" several of the main symptoms in the "Present Illness," asking if the patient is different from his usual self with respect to these symptoms.

Patient's account:

Informant's account:

Medical History

Birth and development (Specify when information is from "baby book" recorded at time of event.)

City of birth:

Hospital where born:

Complications during mother's pregnancy (illness, drugs, injuries, etc.):

Complications at birth (prematurity, Cesarean section, cyanosis, birth injury, etc.):

Include all injuries and illnesses recalled.

Injuries later in infancy, childhood or adolescence. Age of each injury, symptoms, treatment, duration, and outcome. Emotional significance? Disability?

Illnesses later in infancy, childhood or adolescence. Age of each illness, symptoms, treatment, duration, and outcome. Emotional significance? Disability?

Have you seen doctors in their offices for any other reasons? Age, symptoms, treatment, duration, and outcome. Emotional significance? Disability?

At what age did menstrual periods start?

Scholastic History

Patient's and parents' information about school.

Tell me all the schools you have attended:

Name of school and city:

Calendar years in each school:

Grades attended in each school:

General performance:

Inclusive dates of school absences:

Reasons for each period of absence:

Objective school record (record here *only* information from schools.)

Name of school and city:

Dates in each school:

Grades attended:

Intellegence Quotient:

Academic record and remarks:

Were you (was he or she):

Ever expelled or suspended from school?
What ages and grades?
What reasons?
Ever truant on the average of more than once a year?
What ages and grades?
What reasons?
Ever in fights leading to trouble with school authorities?
What ages and grades?
What reasons?
Ever failed in a subject?
What ages and grades?
What reasons?
Ever made to repeat a semester or a year?
What ages and grades?
What reasons?
Ever miss most of a semester or year because of illness; because of any reason?
What ages and grades?
What reasons?

What are your major interests in school (academic interests, athletic, etc.)?
Specify type of interest, performance, extent of involvement:
What are your major interests outside school (hobbies, etc.)?
Specify type of interest, performance, extent of involvement:

Personal Relationships

How have you (he or she) gotten along with:
Schoolmates?
Other friends?
Teachers?
Other people (specify)?

Parental Home

Tell me about your parents (and step or foster parents if applicable). What are (or were) they like? How have you gotten along with them?
Were your parents ever divorced?
When?
What do you remember about this and the effect it had on you?
Were your parents ever separated?
When? Name each occasion:
What do you remember about this (these times) and the effect on you?

How many brothers and sisters do you have?

(List by name all siblings alive in patient's lifetime with current age. If dead specify age and calendar year of death. List patient and his age in proper sequence, also.)

What is each of them like and how do you get along with them?

Bereavement

Have you lost a parent, brother or sister?

When did he (she or they) die?

What effect did his (or her) death have on you? (List each person, age of patient at time of death and his statement about the effect of this.)

Separation

Have you *ever* been separated from either parent for more than two months for any reason, *including* being away at school or camp?

Age of separation:

Parent from whom separated:

Length of separation:

Reason for separation:

Parental Deviance

Was either of your parents:

Jailed?

Which parent?

Inclusive dates:

Details:

Not a steady worker:

Which parent?

Inclusive dates:

Details: (Specify exactly how not steady and consequences to person and family.)

A heavy drinker?

Which parent?

Inclusive dates:

Details: (Specify amount, duration and consequences of drinking to drinker and family.)

Family's Occupation

Father's current employer:

Father's current specific job:

Length of time father working for this employer:
Total earnings of father last year:
Mother's current employer:
Mother's current specific job:
Length of time mother working for this employer:
Total earnings of mother last year:
Current employer of other main family wage earner (specify relationship):
Other wage earner's current specific job:
Length of time other wage earner working for this employer:
Total earnings of other wage earner last year:

Legal Problems

Have you ever been arrested for any reason (including while you were in service)?
Have you ever been in prison or detention for any reason (including while you were in service)?
Age of arrest:
Offense:
Length of time in prison or detention:
Circumstances of release (parole, etc.):

Military History

Have you ever been in military service?
Branch of service:
Age of enlistment or draft:
Length of time in service:
Last rank held:
Reason for discharge:

Hospitalization

Have you ever been a patient in a hospital before, for any reason?
Inclusive dates:
Name and place of hospital:
Reason for hospitalization:
Treatment:
Outcome:
Doctor's name:

Family Psychiatric History

Has anyone related to you ever been a patient in a mental hospital or ever had trouble with nervousness, depression, nervous breakdown, heavy drinking, including your parents, brothers, sisters, uncles, aunts, cousins, grandparents (and children, if any)?

Relative:
Symptoms:
Inclusive dates if illness:
Age of relative at onset:
Treatment:
Outcome:

Has anyone related to you ever killed himself, including parents, brothers, sisters, uncles, aunts, cousins, or grandparents?

Relative:
Age of suicide:
Means of suicide:
Evidence of mental illness:

Marital History

Age of marriage(s):
Date(s) of marriage(s):
Inclusive dates of separation:
Reasons for separation:
Date of divorce:
Date of spouse's death:

Job History

What is your job now?
Job history. List most recent job first.

Type of job:
Employer:
Inclusive dates held:
Why left that job?
Patient's own gross income per year:
Actual time not working (dates):
Reason not working (include symptoms):

How much money per year has your family made this past year before taxes (total income parents *or* of patient and spouse plus any other source of money):

Have you ever had personal difficulties with employers, subordinates, or fellow workers on any job?

When (which job)?
Why?

Immediate Family

Can you tell me approximately the years in which the (his, her) members of your immediate family were born? Spouse, mother, father, all sibs, all children, stepparents. Specify if parents adoptive or step. Have you lost any members of your immediate family?

Relative, including spouse:

Year of birth (exact date if in the past year):

Year of death (exact date if in past year):

Cause of death:

Symptom Inventory

General criteria for scoring a symptom as positive:

A. The symptom led the patient to go to a physician.

B. The symptom was disabling, causing some degree of change in the patient's life.

C. The symptom led the patient on more than one occasion to take medication.

D. The physician believes because of its clinical importance the symptom should be scored as positive even though it does not fulfill criteria A, B, or C. For example, a spell of blindness lasting a few minutes which the patient may minimize, *i.e.,* deny that criteria A through C apply, would be scored as positive. This criterion is also meant to include any symptom that the physician believes to be of clinical significance to him, without regard to its fulfilling criteria A, B, or C. When this criterion is used, mark the item "D."

E. A symptom is *not* scored if it is explainable by known somatic disease of the patient, unless such explanation is recorded in interview.

General instructions for recording responses to each symptom:

(1) Any positive response must be elaborated with regard to its *qualitative description,* its *frequency,* and its *chronology.*

(2) Any positive response requires a statement as to whether associated with present illness.

(3) Any response to which the patient gives a tentative positive response but which is scored as negative must be elaborated.

__1. Nervousness (If yes, ask patient what "nervousness" is like for him and describe.)

__2. a. Short of breath

__ b. Heart pounding

__ c. Chest pain

__ d. Anxiety attacks

__ e. Dizziness

__3. Headache

__4. a. Easily tired

__ b. Weakness

__5. a. Blind
__ b. Other trouble with vision (blurring, spots, diplopia, "tunnel")
__ c. Loss of ability to feel over any part of body
__ d. Paralyzed, all or any part of body
__ e. Deaf
__ f. Loss of voice
__ g. Lump in throat
__ h. Fainting
__6. a. Abdominal pain
__ b. Abdominal bloating or gas
__ c. Constipation
__ d. Diarrhea
__ e. Unable to control bowels
__ f. Nauseated
__ g. Vomiting
__7. a. Painful urination
__ b. Unable to urinate
__ c. Unable to control urine
__ d. Wetting the bed
__8. a. Tics
__ b. Obsessions
__ c. Compulsions
__ d. Fears
__9. a. Back pain
__ b. Pain in arms or legs
__ c. Any other pain
__10. a. Irregular menstrual periods
__ b. Pain with periods
__ c. Tense or depressed or nervous before, during, or after periods
__ d. Heavy bleeding during periods
__11. Ever pregnant
__12. a. Pain on sexual intercourse
__ b. Failure to reach climax
__ c. Unable to get erection
__ d. Other problems with sex
__ e. Unfaithful to husband or wife
__13. Unconscious for any reason
__14. Convulsions of any type
__15. a. Running away from school or home
__ b. Wandering from place to place
__16. a. Arguing

___ b. Fighting, or hitting people
___ c. Temper outbursts
___ d. Damaging or tearing up things
___ e. Cruel to children or animals
___ f. Setting fires
___17. a. Lying
___ b. Stealing
___ c. Cheating
___18. a. Depressed, sad, blue, etc.
___ b. Crying
___ c. Felt life was hopeless
___ d. Felt you were hopelessly sick or mixed up
___ e. Worrying more than usual
___19. a. Felt guilty
___ b. Felt undeserving or worthless
___ c. Felt a burden to others
___20. a. Wanted to die
___ b. Talked or wrote of killing yourself
___ c. Thought of killing yourself
___ d. Tried to kill yourself
___ e. Thought of killing anybody else
___ f. Talked of killing anybody else
___ g. Tried to kill anybody
___21. a. Loss of interest in activities or less activity than formerly
___ b. Temporarily unable or unwilling to work at school or job
___ c. Not keep self clean or well groomed
___22. a. Trouble getting to sleep
___ b. Restless sleep
___ c. Waking up and not being able to go back to sleep
___23. a. Trouble thinking or concentrating (describe)
___ b. Trouble with memory
___24. a. Lost appetite
___ b. Increased appetite
___ c. Lost weight
___ d. Gained weight
___25. a. Thoughts fast
___ b. Talking a lot
___ c. Less need for sleep
___ d. Increased libido
___26. a. Elated, high (when not taking drugs or alcohol)
___ b. Felt especially strong or powerful or important
___ c. Special mission (*e.g.*, religious, political, etc.)
___ d. Talking with God, messages from God, etc.

__ e. Other grandiose ideas or plans
__27. a. People watching or talking about you
__ b. People following you
__ c. People making plans for or against you
__28. a. People reading your mind
__ b. People controlling your thoughts or actions
__ c. Influences or messages from other or from T.V., radio, etc.
__29. a. Felt unreal
__ b. Things seem changed
__ c. Are you changing?
__ d. Are you mixed up by what is going on?
__30. a. Hear noises or voices or own thoughts
__ b. See visions on other things
__ c. Smell unusual or peculiar smells
__ d. Peculiar feelings or sensations anywhere in body

Alcohol

__1. Do you drink alcohol in any form?
__2. How frequently do you drink? (Times/month)
__3. Amount in ounces per week expressed as whiskey (1 oz. whiskey = 3 oz. wine = 8 oz. beer)
__4. Has your family ever objected to your drinking?
__5. Did you ever think you drank too much?
__6. Do others think you drink too much for your own good?
__7. Guilty about drinking?
__8. Ever lost friends because of drinking?
__9. Did you ever get into trouble at school or work because of drinking?
__10. Did you ever lose a job on account of drinking?
__11. Did you ever have trouble with auto driving (speeding, accident, etc.) because of drinking?
__12. Have you ever been arrested, even for a few hours, because of drinking and/or disturbing the peace?
__13. Fighting when drinking?
__14. Have you ever gone on benders? (48 hours of drinking associated with default of usual obligations; must have occurred more than once. There must be repetitive drinking bouts of at least 48 hours if no obligations are defaulted, *i.e.*, while on leave from military service.)
__15. Ever wanted to stop drinking and couldn't?
__16. Ever tried to drink only under certain circumstances (time of day, places, associates)?

__17. Ever drink before breakfast?
__18. Drinking unusual things such as hair tonic, paint solvent, rubbing alcohol?
__19. "Blackouts" (loss of memory) with drinking?
__20. Impotence?
__21. DT's, other complications (cirrhosis, hallucinosis, tremulousness, shakes, etc.)?
__22. Fearful when drinking?
__23. Age started heavy drinking.
__24. Age stopped heavy drinking.
__25. Evaluation of alcoholic status:
  __ Chronic alcoholic, active
  __ Chronic alcoholic, in remission
  __ Heavy drinker
  __ Mild drinker (normal social drinking)
  __ Teetotaler

Drugs

__1. Do you ever take drugs for sleeping?
__2. Every night?
__3. During the day?
__4. Do you ever take tranquilizers or nerve medicine?
__5. Have you ever used other drugs? (Specify marijuana, the common hallucinogens, amphetamines, sedatives, etc., or the various slang terms for these substances.)
__6. Do you think you ever took too many drugs?
__7. Did you ever want to stop taking drugs and couldn't?
__8. Were you ever addicted to any drugs?
__9. Evaluation of drug status:
  __ Addict
  __ Took too many
  __ Took occasionally (excludes prescribed medication)
  __ None

Sexual History

At what age did you start dating?
How often have you dated this past year?
Have you ever gone steady or been engaged?
  Specify number of times and inclusive ages:
Have you ever had sexual relations (with a member of the opposite sex)?
  Age of first experience:

Total number of partners:
Frequency of sexual relations:
Sexual relations (with member of the same sex):
Age of first experience:
Total number of partners:
Frequency of sexual relations:

Suicide Communication (ask patient and informant separately)

Have you (has he or she) ever talked to anyone about
__a. Wanting to die
—b. Being better off dead; tired of living
—c. Others (or his family) being better off if you were dead
__d. Committing suicide
__e. Any similar ideas
__f. Have you (he, she) made actual suicide attempts?
__g. References to methods of committing suicide
__h. Dire predictions
"I won't be here tomorrow." "You'll find a dead man in the streets." "I am going to (or wish to) get off the face of the earth." "Someday you'll find me dead." "This is your last kiss." "This is the last time I will see you." "I won't be here (at some future date)." "If something happens to me don't be surprised."
__i. References to dying before or with relative or friend
__j. Putting affairs in order or planning to
__k. Can't take it any longer; no other way out
__l. References to burial or grave
__m. Statement of being afraid or not being afraid to die
__n. Talk about suicides of other
—o. Not buying new things
__p. Taunts and threats
__q. Other
"I'm going to throw everything in your lap." "What would you do without me?" "I'm not responsible for what I do."

For each type of communication, specify:
Dates when (inclusive dates if over period of time):
To whom:
Frequency:
Drinking? Drugs?
Other circumstances and details, etc:

Mental Status

A. General appearance and behavior:
B. Speech:

C. Mood:
D. Content of thought: (Describe anything not described under the history.)
E. Orientation:
   __1. Time
   __2. Place
   __3. Person
F. Memory:
G. Intellectual function:
H. Insight and judgment:

Appendix II
Diagnostic criteria

Depression

1. An onset, whether rapid or gradual, after which there is a difference from usual self, manifested predominantly by a dysphoric mood.

2. The change includes at least two of the following symptoms: self-blaming or self-negating attitude, diminished interest, excessive worrying, death wishes.

3. The change includes at least four of the following symptoms: anorexia, insomnia, decreased libido, tired, trouble thinking or concentrating, diminished or impaired activity, not keeping self well groomed, crying, or other agitated behavior.

4. No disturbance of consciousness.

5. No other diagnosis likely to explain symptoms.

Mania

1. An onset, whether rapid or gradual, after which there is a difference from usual self, predominantly manifested by a euphoric or frantic mood.

2. The change includes at least two of the following symptoms: inappropriately elated reaction to events, grandiose ideas about self, extreme impatience with restraint, excessive plans, excessive desire to spend money.

3. The change includes at least two of the following symptoms: overtalkativeness, thinking faster or changing subject rapidly, increased energy or physical activity, less sleep.

4. No disturbance of consciousness.

5. No other diagnosis likely to explain symptoms.

Schizophrenia

1. An impairing psychiatric illness which is a change from previous state, which cannot be accounted for on the basis of organic brain disease, and in which symptoms or disability have persisted

since onset, although the longitudinal course may be characterized by great changes in the severity of the disability.

2. A persistent disorder of the form of thought (*e.g.*, concept formation, comprehension, or association), or at least two of the following: perceptual disturbance (for example, hallucinations), thought content disturbance, and ideas of passivity.

3. Blunted or incongruous affect.

4. Bizarre or withdrawn behavior.

5. No other diagnosis more likely.

Antisocial Personality (adapted from Robins[1])

A chronic disorder with at least four of the following symptoms:

1. School problems: recurrent truancy, suspensions or expulsions for misbehavior, fighting.
2. Poor work history (if not in school): firings, quitting jobs with no other jobs available, personality conflicts, or fights at work.
3. Excessive drug use, with social, scholastic, or work impairment.
4. Excessive alcohol use, with social, scholastic, or work impairment.
5. Arrests: three or more non-traffic arrests.
6. Habitual physical aggressiveness.
7. Sexual promiscuity or perversion.
8. Suicidal attempts.
9. Habitually impulsive behavior.
10. Vagrancy.
11. Many somatic symptoms.
12. Habitual lying.
13. Few friends.
14. Use of aliases (to conceal identity, not as a joke).
15. Lack of guilt.

Hysteria (adapted from Perley and Guze[2])

1. A chronic or recurrent illness, presenting with a dramatic, vague, or complicated medical history.

2. At least 25 medically unexplained symptoms in at least nine of the following groups:

Group 1
Headaches
Sickly majority of life

Group 2
Blindness

Paralysis
Anesthesia
Aphonia
Fits or convulsions
Unconsciousness
Amnesia
Deafness
Hallucinations
Urinary retention
Trouble walking
Other unexplained "neurologic" symptoms

Group 3

Fatigue
Lump in throat
Fainting spells
Visual blurring
Weakness
Dysuria

Group 4

Breathing difficulty
Palpitation
Anxiety attacks
Chest pain
Dizziness

Group 5

Anorexia
Weight loss
Marked fluctuations in weight
Nausea
Abdominal bloating
Food intolerances
Diarrhea
Constipation

Group 6

Abdominal pain
Vomiting

Group 7

Dysmenorrhea
Menstrual irregularity
Amenorrhea
Excessive bleeding

Group 8

Sexual indifference
Frigidity

Dyspareunia
Other sexual difficulties
Vomiting all nine months of pregnancy at least once, or hospitalization for hyperemesis gravidarum

Group 9

Back pain
Joint pain
Extremity pain
Burning pains of the sexual organs, mouth, or rectum
Other bodily pains

Group 10

Nervousness
Fears
Depressed feelings
Need to quit working, or inability to carry on regular duties because of feeling sick
Crying easily
Feeling life is hopeless
Thinking a good deal about dying
Wanting to die
Thinking about suicide
Suicide attempts

Anxiety Neurosis (adapted from Feighner, *et al.*[3])

1. Chronic nervousness with recurrent anxiety attacks manifested by apprehension, fearfulness, or sense of impending doom, with at least four of the following symptoms present during the majority of attacks: (a) dyspnea, (b) palpitations, (c) chest pain or discomfort, (d) choking or smothering sensation, (e) dizziness, and (f) paresthesias.

2. The anxiety attacks are essential to the diagnosis and must occur at times other than marked physical exertion of life-threatening situations, and in the absence of medical illness that *could* account for symptoms of anxiety. There must have been at least six anxiety attacks, each separated by at least a week from the others.

3. In the presence of other psychiatric illness(es) this diagnosis is made *only* if the criteria described in 1 and 2 antedate the onset of the other psychiatric illness by at least two years.

Obsessive Compulsive Neurosis (adapted from Feighner, *et al.*[3])

1. Obsessions or compulsions are the dominant symptoms. They are defined as recurrent or persistent ideas, thoughts, images, feelings, impulses, or movements, which must be accompanied by a

sense of subjective compulsion and a desire to resist the event, the event being recognized by the individual as foreign to his personality or nature, *i.e.,* "ego-alien."

2. Patients with primary or probable primary affective disorder, or with schizophrenia or probable schizophrenia, who manifest obsessive-compulsive features, do not receive the additional diagnosis of obsessive compulsive neurosis.

Phobic Neurosis (adapted from Feighner, *et al.*[3])

1. Phobias are the dominant symptoms. They are defined as persistent and recurring fears which the patient tries to resist or avoid and at the same time considers unreasonable.

2. Symptoms of anxiety, tension, nervousness, and depression may accompany the phobias; however, patients with another definable psychiatric illness should not receive the additional diagnosis of phobic neurosis.

Anorexia Nervosa (adapted from Feighner, *et al.*[3])

1. Anorexia with accompanying weight loss of at least 25% of original body weight.

2. A distorted, implacable attitude towards eating, food, or weight that overrides hunger, admonitions, reassurance, and threats, *e.g.,* (a) denial of illness with a failure to recognize nutritional needs, (b) apparent enjoyment in losing weight with overt manifestation that food refusal is a pleasurable indulgence, (c) a desired body image of extreme thinness with overt evidence that it is rewarding to the patient to achieve and maintain this state, and (d) unusual hoarding or handling of food.

3. No known medical illness that could account for the anorexia and weight loss.

4. No other known psychiatric disorder, with particular reference to primary affective disorders, schizophrenia, obsessive compulsive and phobic neurosis. (The assumption is made that even though it may appear phobic or obsessional, food refusal alone is not sufficient to qualify for obsessive compulsive or phobic disease.)

5. At least two of the following manifestations. (a) Amenorrhea. (b) Lanugo. (c) Bradycardia (persistent resting pulse of 60 or less). (d) Periods of overactivity. (e) Episodes of bulimia. (f) Vomiting (may be self-induced).

Organic Brain Syndrome (adapted from Feighner, *et al.*[3])

This diagnosis is made when *either* criterion 1 or criterion 2 is present.

1. Two of the following manifestations must be present (in the presence of muteness the diagnosis must be deferred.) (a) Impairment of orientation. (b) Impairment of memory. (c) Deterioration of other intellectual functions.

2. This diagnosis is also made if the patient has at least one manifestation (1) in addition to a known probable cause for organic brain syndrome.

Mental Retardation (identical to criteria of Feighner, *et al.*[3])

This disorder, which has different causes, is described both in terms of intellectual impairment and social maladaption in DSM-II. In view of the fact that the social adaptation scales have not been standardized to the level of current intelligence tests, only the latter are used in making this diagnosis. The following criteria are used:

1. When the I.Q. is available from currently acceptable tests, the categories of DSM-II are used.

2. In the absence of I.Q. tests, the following will be accepted as evidence of suspected mental retardation: (a) Despite continued effort, an individual fails the same grade two years in succession, or (b) despite continued effort, the individual fails to pass the sixth grade by the time he is 16 years old.

(Caution should be used in making the diagnosis of mental retardation in the presence of another psychiatric illness, *i.e.,* schizophrenia, severe affective disorders, antisocial personality disorder.)

Alcoholism

All three criteria must be present:

1. History of at least one year's duration, with chronicity.

2. Patient or informant says patient drinks too much; or intoxication more than twice a week; or history of withdrawal symptoms (tremulousness, convulsions, delirium tremens).

3. Social, scholastic, job, or legal problems related to alcohol abuse.

Drug Abuse

All three criteria must be present:

1. History of at least one year's duration, with chronicity.

2. Patient or informant says patient abuses drugs; or history of illegal sources; or history of abuse of legal sources; or frequent intoxication; or withdrawal symptoms.

3. Social, scholastic, job, or legal problems related to excessive drug use.

Homosexuality

Persistent homoerotic feelings and homosexual activity, regardless of whether heterosexual activity is also present. Transient experimentation in pre-teens or early teenage years (*i.e.*, mutual masturbation) is not sufficient to qualify an adolescent for this diagnosis.

REFERENCES

1. Robins, L. N. *Deviant Children Grown Up: A Sociological and Psychiatric Study of Sociopathic Personality*. Baltimore, Williams and Wilkins Company, 1966.
2. Perley, M. J., and Guze, S. B. Hysteria—the stability and usefulness of clinical criteria: a quantitative study based on a follow-up period of 6–8 years in 39 patients. N. Engl. J. Med. *266:* 421–426, 1962.
3. Feighner, J. P., Robins, E., Guze, S. B., Woodruff, R. A., Winokur, G., and Munoz, R. Diagnostic criteria for use in psychiatric research. Arch. Gen. Psychiatry *26:* 57–63, 1972.

Index